AF587112

OVERCOMING HEARING LOSS

From Drug Therapy to Cochlear Implant Surgery

Latest Advancements in the Management of Hearing Loss

OVERCOMING HEARING LOSS

From Drug Therapy to Cochlear Implant Surgery

Latest Advancements in the Management of Hearing Loss

Adrien A. Eshraghi, MD, MSc, FACS
University of Miami, USA

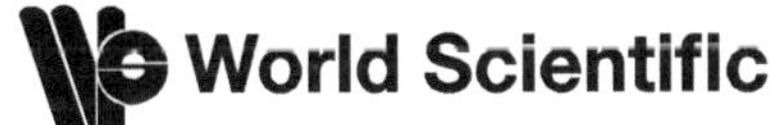

NEW JERSEY • LONDON • SINGAPORE • BEIJING • SHANGHAI • HONG KONG • TAIPEI • CHENNAI • TOKYO

Published by

World Scientific Publishing Co. Pte. Ltd.
5 Toh Tuck Link, Singapore 596224
USA office: 27 Warren Street, Suite 401-402, Hackensack, NJ 07601
UK office: 57 Shelton Street, Covent Garden, London WC2H 9HE

British Library Cataloguing-in-Publication Data
A catalogue record for this book is available from the British Library.

We would like to acknowledge both Western University in Canada (Dr. Ladak and Dr. Agrawal) and Uppsala University in Sweden (Dr. Li and Dr. Rask-Andersen) for the cover photo representing a cochlea implanted by a cochlear implant electrode. Their research teams used a novel technique involving a massive synchrotron particle accelerator to create imaging of intact cochlear micro-anatomy with unprecedented detail. (permission was obtained by MED-EL Corporation to show their electrode within the cochlea)

OVERCOMING HEARING LOSS: FROM DRUG THERAPY TO COCHLEAR IMPLANT SURGERY
Latest Advancements in the Management of Hearing Loss

Copyright © 2024 by World Scientific Publishing Co. Pte. Ltd.

All rights reserved. This book, or parts thereof, may not be reproduced in any form or by any means, electronic or mechanical, including photocopying, recording or any information storage and retrieval system now known or to be invented, without written permission from the publisher.

For photocopying of material in this volume, please pay a copying fee through the Copyright Clearance Center, Inc., 222 Rosewood Drive, Danvers, MA 01923, USA. In this case permission to photocopy is not required from the publisher.

ISBN 978-981-12-8796-1 (hardcover)
ISBN 978-981-12-8850-0 (paperback)
ISBN 978-981-12-8797-8 (ebook for institutions)
ISBN 978-981-12-8798-5 (ebook for individuals)

For any available supplementary material, please visit
https://www.worldscientific.com/worldscibooks/10.1142/13723#t=suppl

Foreword

In an era where the intricacies of human health are increasingly understood, this timely tome emerges as an invaluable resource for those touched by the silent tide of hearing loss. It offers relevant history and an explanatory overview of the human ear's delicate architecture and the multifaceted causes of auditory impairments, providing a lighthouse of knowledge accessible to patients and practitioners alike.

This work is an amalgamation of the scientific rigor and compassionate insight of esteemed experts who paint a comprehensive picture of the auditory system's magnificence and its vulnerabilities. From the molecular dance within the cochlea to the socio-economic ripples of hearing loss, the breadth of discussion presented here is as deep as it is wide.

Beyond a mere aggregation of facts, this book stands as a testament to the resilience of individuals facing auditory challenges and the relentless pursuit of innovation and excellence in auditory healthcare. It weaves together narratives of scientific discovery, clinical wisdom, and the lived experiences of patients into a fabric that comforts and educates.

As you delve into the ensuing chapters, you will find yourself on a journey through the corridors of cutting-edge research, clinical anecdotes, and heartfelt stories that underscore the significance of our auditory connection to the world. This book does not just inform; it transforms understanding into action and challenges into hope. It demonstrates how near the field is to a quantum leap into genetic and cell treatments.

With each chapter, may you gain a deeper appreciation for the significance of human communication and the strength of the human spirit to overcome. Here's to the symphony of life that awaits within these pages and to the wisdom of those who have contributed so ably.

D. Bradley Welling, MD, PhD
Walter Augustus Lecompte Distinguished Professor
Harvard Department of Otolaryngology Head & Neck Surgery
Massachusetts Eye and Ear Infirmary
Massachusetts General Hospital

Preface

Hearing loss affects millions of individuals worldwide and is one of the most common and impactful sensory deficits affecting humans. It impacts not only the affected individuals hearing but also their overall quality of life, it is also associated with comorbidities such as dementia and depression as well as increased risk of falls. All these secondary effects also negatively impact the patient's quality of life.

Hearing loss affects people of all ages and demographics for a plethora of reasons including but not limited to aging, drug side effects, genetic causes, noise trauma, and infections. There are a wide variety of treatments for hearing loss ranging from medications to implantable hearing devices. With this area of medicine being very specialized and rapidly advancing it can be difficult for healthcare professionals to stay informed of the treatments available for their patients. Patients can utilize this book to be informed and participate actively in their own care with their healthcare provider. In this book, *Overcoming Hearing Loss: From Drug Therapy to Cochlear Implant Surgery*, expert physicians, surgeons, and scientists have worked to compile and describe the pathophysiology and etiology of hearing loss as well as the most current treatment modalities available for individuals having hearing loss of any severity or origin.

Each chapter stands independent, begins with a short summary of its contents followed by a comprehensive review of the given topic, and concludes with complete list of relevant citations. Each chapter may have accompanying figures and tables displaying the data in condense form for easy reading. This book is intended to be an overview of hearing loss and the most current therapies available for those at all levels including patients, medical students, audiologists, researchers, and physicians from all fields.

The first chapter explores the anatomy and pathophysiology of the ear. This chapter gives a clear overview of the anatomy and physiology of the hearing system which will allow for a better understanding of the various forms of hearing loss and their treatments. It delves into the basic anatomy of the hearing apparatus and how these sensory areas change in relation to hearing loss.

The second chapter discusses the various etiologies of sensorineural hearing loss. A diagnosis of hearing loss is the first step in the process of understanding and treating a patient's change in hearing. The diagnostic process and the criteria for the various levels of hearing loss are discussed in further detail. In addition to discussing the causes of hearing loss, the consequences of those living with uncorrected hearing loss, including increased risk of dementia, delirium, falls, and mortality are reviewed.

There are many causes of hearing loss, some are less avoidable, such as aging, genetic diseases, and ototoxic medications. However, there are some associated correlations with hearing loss that are preventable including exposure to loud environments and smoking. The third chapter discusses the primary and secondary prevention of hearing loss. The causes of hearing loss that are preventable as well as the most appropriate current preventative measures are reviewed in this chapter.

Genetic testing is a quickly growing practice in every field of medicine. It can reliably and quickly show possible molecular links for any disease or symptom being examined. Genetic links within hearing loss are discussed in the fourth chapter. The most frequently implicated genes in hearing loss are presented as well as the most commonly used genetic testing methods. Multigene testing is a commonly utilized method which is required due to the vast number of involved genes in hearing loss. The effects of known genetic differences as the etiology of hearing loss on prognosis, recurrence, evaluation, and ultimately treatment are examined. Understanding this important information in relation to hearing loss will allow for a better understanding of more targeted therapies for these patients as well as underscore the need for evidence-based algorithms to more accurately diagnose and treat hearing loss.

There are three general categories of hearing loss: sensorineural, conductive, and mixed hearing loss. The fifth chapter delves into both conductive and mixed hearing loss, with the goal of presenting the differences and similarities in the causes, diagnosis, and the treatment between these two forms of hearing loss. The various etiologies and managements are discussed based on the portion of the ear that they affect; external, middle, or inner ear. When diagnosing hearing loss, it is imperative to understand the root anatomical or physiologic causes of the hearing loss so it can be appropriately managed by a clinician or surgeon.

Chapter six discusses the causes as well as the most current and promising medical treatments for the various forms of sensorineural hearing loss (SNHL), which includes presbycusis, noise induced hearing loss, and sudden SNHL. Sensorineural hearing loss involves deficit either the cochlea, the cochlear nerve, or the brain. This form of hearing loss has treatments that range from medications targeting the underlying mechanism, such as steroids and immunological agents, to hearing aids or cochlear implants to help the patient regain some or all of their hearing.

Hearing loss may be associated with other symptoms depending on the underlying mechanism. Two of the most distressing associated symptoms are tinnitus (ringing in the ears) and hyperacusis. These two symptoms are a great challenge to professionals as they have variable diagnostic testing results and few effective and long-term treatments. The seventh chapter is an overview of tinnitus and hyperacusis as well as a discussion of the current best practices in their management and treatment.

Immunological causes of hearing loss are varied, but are hallmarked by new onset asymmetric sensorineural hearing loss and are traditionally treated with corticosteroids. However, many patients remain unresponsive to this therapy and will require newer more targeted therapies. The eighth chapter reviews novel immunologic-related approaches to the treatment of sensorineural hearing loss. This chapter delves into the causes of hearing loss that are most responsive to immunological treatments as well as the diagnosis, benefits and the disadvantages of this line of treatment.

Medical devices have been a hallmark of the treatment of hearing loss since their creation in the 18th century, with the introduction of the ear trumpet. In the more than 300 years since this, many new and cutting-edge tools have been developed. The ninth chapter discusses the most current medical devices for hearing loss including traditional hearing aids, bone anchored hearing aids, cochlear implants, and brain stem implants. Each device group is discussed in detail including the indications, contraindications, implementation process and outcomes for each device.

Cochlear implants have been the gold standard to provide auditory rehabilitation to the individuals with profound sensorineural hearing loss since their inception. They are the first implantable devices that can restore one of the human senses. There are many different types of cochlear implants, which differ in the types and numbers of electrodes as well as the type and capabilities of the associated processor. The tenth chapter delves into a comprehensive discussion of cochlear implants including their history, mechanism of action, indications, surgical implantation, activation, current applications, and future perspectives. With significant improvement in this technology, their indication is expanding significantly, helping more and more patients to be able to hear again.

Single sided deafness involves asymmetrical hearing loss and is associated with a plethora of negative impacts on the patient such as poor language skills, inability to locate sound, and poor hearing in noisy environments. The eleventh chapter discusses single sided deafness, delving into the impacts and management of this type of hearing loss that interferes with sound localization and affects quality of life of many patients. The etiologies of single sided deafness as well as the various treatment modalities to restore as much hearing and function as possible are discussed.

The twelfth chapter discusses the current state of medical management for auditory disorders and future perspectives for treatment. In the past, there were limited modalities of treatment for hearing loss, particularly when it comes to medical management. Historically, corticosteroids alone were the only medication to manage sensorineural hearing loss. More recently, research groups are making significant advances in this field to discover more efficacious drugs for this patient population. The advances and challenges of gene therapy for hearing loss and balance disorders are presented and discussed by the experts in the chapter thirteen.

Chapter fourteen discusses the use of robots in otologic surgery in the treatment of hearing loss. This is a new and rapidly progressing field of otolaryngology. This chapter discusses the varying levels of robotic assistance such as assistive, teleoperated, and autonomous in two of the most impacted areas of otologic surgery; drilling the mastoid bone and electrode insertion during cochlea implantation. Both of these maneuvers require precise movement by the surgeon and have negative implications for the recipient if done incorrectly.

The last chapter discusses how to advocate for one's rights as a child or an adult with hearing loss. It is written by a patient with hearing loss who is a successful and strong advocate for appropriately managing hearing loss. Proactively tackling one's hearing loss or supporting a child along his journey begins with pursuing hearing technology or other therapies that are appropriate and available. Self-advocacy also means we recognize that hearing loss often changes over time, just as one's life circumstances change over time. Recognizing that there is a continuum of hearing care solutions and staying abreast of information that can help someone pursue the right solution is critical to the partnership between patients and hearing care providers. This chapter provides encouragement to practice self-advocacy to benefit from the wide-ranging laws that may exist today and provide opportunities that can help children and adults to take advantage of all that life has to offer.

I would like to take a moment to thank the incredible contributors and experts that accepted the opportunity to create this comprehensive book to help guide patients and professionals from all areas of life on the current state of hearing loss and its treatment. Their hours of tireless work and contributions allowed this book to be a comprehensive and informative resource in an easy-to-read compilation. I would like to give a special thanks to my neurotologists colleagues, audiologists, fellows, residents, and students at University of Miami Ear Institute that enriched my experience in caring for patients with hearing loss over the last 20 years; and recognize, especially, my collaborators at the University of Miami Hearing Research and the Cochlear Implant Laboratory at UM for their constant support and invaluable input in creating this book. Lastly, I'd like to thank you, the reader, for embarking on this journey with us.

Adrien A. Eshraghi, MD, MSc, FACS
Professor of Otolaryngology, Neurosurgery, Pediatrics,
and Biomedical Engineering
UHealth - University of Miami Health System
Jackson Memorial Hospital
University of Miami Miller School of Medicine

Contents

List of Corresponding Authors

Joe Walter Kutz Jr., MD, FACS, Professor of Otolaryngology and Neurological Surgery at The University of Texas Southwestern Medical Center, Department of Otolaryngology, The University of Texas Southwestern Medical Center, Dallas, TX, United States; Department of Neurological Surgery, The University of Texas Southwestern Medical Center, Dallas, TX, USA.

Brandon Isaacson, MD, FACS, Professor of Otolaryngology and Neurological Surgery at The University of Texas Southwestern Medical Center, Department of Otolaryngology, The University of Texas Southwestern Medical Center, Dallas, TX, United States; Department of Neurological Surgery, The University of Texas Southwestern Medical Center, Dallas, TX, USA.

Adrien A. Eshraghi MD, MSc, FACS, Professor of Otolaryngology, Neurosurgery, Pediatrics, and Biomedical Engineering University of Miami, Miller School of Medicine; University of Miami Ear Institute; UHealth - University of Miami Health System; Jackson Memorial Hospital; University of Miami Miller School of Medicine, Miami, Florida, USA.

Michael D. Seidman, MD, FACS, Professor of Otolaryngology and Neurosurgery at the University of Central Florida; University of Central Florida College of Medicine, Orlando, FL, United States.; Otology/Neurotology/Skull Base Surgery Advent Health Celebration, FL, United States.; Medical Wellness Advent Health Celebration, FL, United States.; University of South Florida, Tampa, FL, USA.

A. Eliot Shearer, MD, PhD, Assistant Professor of Otolaryngology Harvard Medical School; Department of Otolaryngology–Head and Neck Surgery, Harvard Medical School, Boston, MA, United States; Department of Otolaryngology and Communication Enhancement, Boston Children's Hospital, Boston, MA, USA.

Ayache Denis, MD, Professor College of Medicine Paris Hospital, Department of Otolaryngology - Head and Neck Surgery, Adolphe de Rothschild Foundation Hospital, Paris, France.

Maria Pia-Tuset, MD, MSc, Chef de Clinic, Department of Otolaryngology — Head and Neck Surgery, Adolphe de Rothschild Foundation Hospital, Paris, France.

Sujana S. Chandrasekhar, MD, FACS, Clinical Professor of Otolaryngology, Zucker School of Medicine at Hofstra-Northwell; Clinical Associate Professor of Otolaryngology at Mount Sinai School of Medicine; Cooperman Barnabas Medical Center, Livingston, NJ; James J. Peters VA Medical Center, The Bronx, NY; Lenox Hill Hospital (Northwell), New York, NY; Manhattan Eye Ear and Throat Hospital (Northwell), New York, NY; New York Eye And Ear Infirmary of Mt. Sinai, Mount Sinai Hospital, New York, NY, USA.

Ali A. Danesh, PhD, Professor, Department of Communication Sciences and Disorders / Communication Disorders Clinic Schmidt College of Medicine, Florida Atlantic University, Boca Raton, FL, USA.

Andrea Vambutas, MD, Professor, Zucker School of Medicine at Hofstra/Northwell, Otolaryngology and Molecular Medicine; Department of Otolaryngology, Donald and Barbara Zucker School of Medicine at Hofstra-Northwell, New Hyde Park, NY, USA.

Oliver F. Adunka MD, MBA, Professor, Department of Otolaryngology at The Ohio State University and Nationwide Children's Hospital; Division of Otology, Neurotology and Cranial Base Surgery, Department of Otolaryngology - Head and Neck Surgery, The Ohio State University Wexner Medical Center, Columbus, OH, USA.

Hillary A. Snapp, PhD, AuD, Professor of Clinical Otolaryngology, Division of Audiology, University of Miami Ear Institute, University of Miami Miller School of Medicine, Miami, FL, USA.

Rahul Mittal, PhD, Scientist, Hearing Research and Cochlear Implant Laboratory, Department of Otolaryngology, University of Miami Miller School of Medicine, Miami, FL, USA.

Aziz El-Amraoui, PhD, Associate Professor Institut Pasteur, Institut de l'Audition, Université Paris Cité, INSERM AO06, Unit Progressive Sensory Disorders, Pathophysiology and Therapy, Paris, France.

Robert F. Labadie MD, PhD, Professor of Otolaryngology, Department of Otolaryngology - Head and Neck Surgery, Medical University of South Carolina, Charleston, SC, USA.

Donna L. Sorkin, MA, Executive Director of the American Cochlear Implant Alliance, Wachington D.C., USA.

1 Anatomy and Physiology of the Inner Ear

Joe Walter Kutz Jr., MD, FACS [1,2];
Brandon Isaacson, MD, FACS[1,2]; Viraj Shah, MD [1,2]

Abstract

The ear is a complex organ which is divided into the outer, middle, and inner ear, consisting of different structures such as external auditory canal, tympanic membrane, ossicles, the cochlea, and vestibular apparatus. These all work in tandem to convert mechanical sound energy into electrical impulses, which are transmitted to the central nervous system. Dissecting deeper into these structures reveals complex electrochemical gradients and molecular processes that help further elucidate the mechanism of hearing and balance function. Patients can experience various symptoms and disorders due to disruptions in the normal functioning of these structures.

For example, damage to the hair cells in the cochlea can result in hearing loss or tinnitus, while damage to the vestibular apparatus can result in dizziness, vertigo, or loss of balance. Understanding the precise mechanisms underlying these disorders is critical for developing effective treatments.

Treatments for inner ear disorders include otoprotective medications, surgical interventions, and physical and vestibular therapy. There are also a variety of devices that can be utilized and implanted to treat both conductive and sensorineural hearing loss (SNHL) such as hearing aids and cochlear implants. Balance therapy and medications can be used to manage vertigo and other balance disorders. Overall, a thorough understanding of inner ear anatomy and physiology is essential for diagnosing and treating disorders affecting this area of the body.

Corresponding Author: Joe Walter Kutz Jr., MD, FACS

[1] Department of Otolaryngology, The University of Texas Southwestern Medical Center, Dallas, TX, United States.

[2] Department of Neurological Surgery, The University of Texas Southwestern Medical Center, Dallas, TX, United States.

Introduction

The inner ear is responsible for the perception of sound, gaze stabilization, and balance (vestibular) function. The cochlea is the portion of the inner ear that converts incoming mechanical sound waves into electrical nerve impulses sent along the auditory nerve to the brain, resulting in hearing perception. In addition, the vestibular end organs of the semicircular canals, utricle, and saccule detect rotational and translational head movements, as well as body position changes relative to gravity. The hearing and vestibular portions of the labyrinth share perilymph and endolymph (inner ear fluids), so inner ear disorders can affect both hearing and balance (Figure 1.1).

The inner ear is referred to as the labyrinth. The bony labyrinth encases the membranous labyrinth and is composed of dense otic capsule bone, including the cochlea, semicircular canals, and the vestibule. The membranous labyrinth is suspended in a fluid known as perilymph, which is nearly identical to cerebrospinal fluid (CSF) and contains high levels of sodium. The membranous labyrinth, which is filled with endolymph fluid,

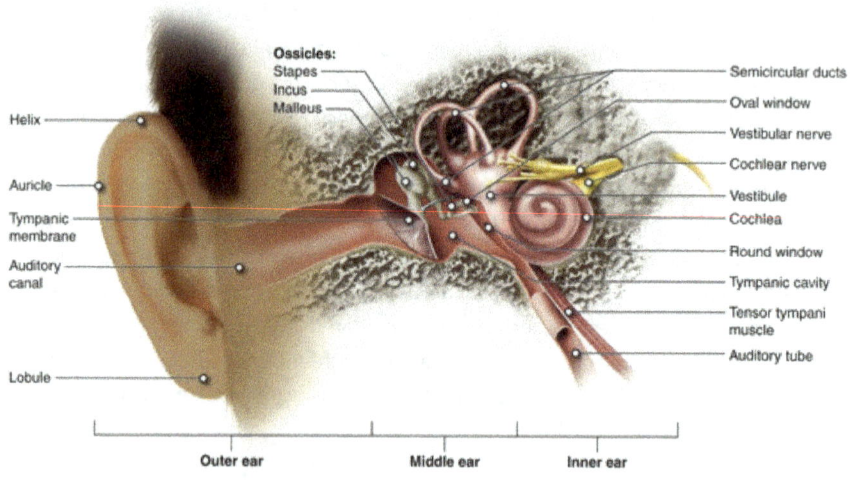

Fig. 1.1 Important structures of the outer, middle, and inner ear.
(**Citation:** Anatomy of the Ear by Cenveo is licensed under CC by-SA 3.0.)

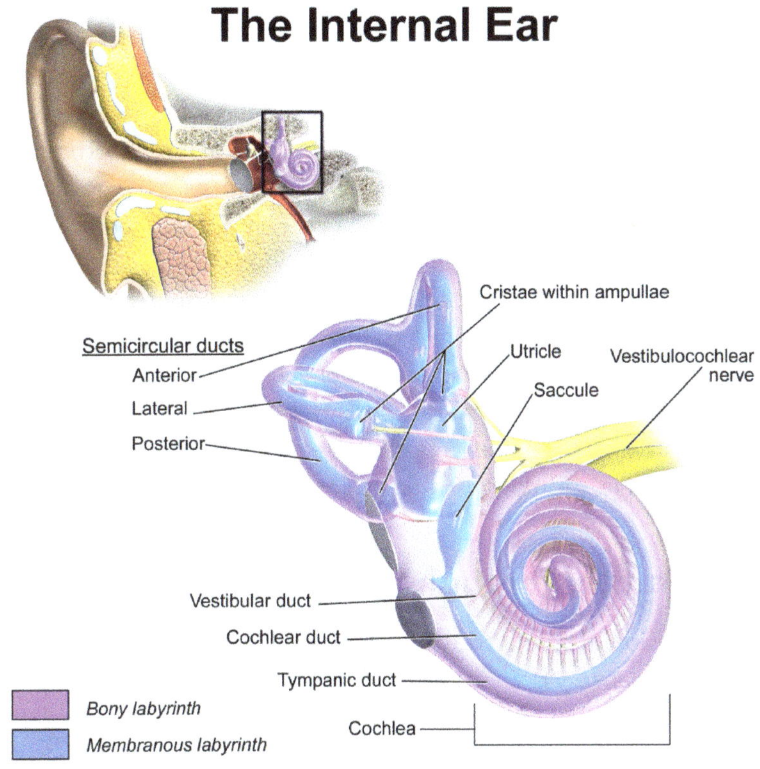

Fig. 1.2 Inner ear anatomy including the cochlea, bony and membranous labyrinth, vestibular apparatus, and vestibulocochlear nerve.

(**Citation:** Blausen.com staff (2014). Medical gallery of Blausen Medical 2014. WikiJournal of Medicine 1 (2). DOI:10.15347/wjm/2014.010. ISSN 2002-4436.)

can be divided into the cochlear duct, semicircular canals, the saccule, utricle, and endolymphatic duct (ELD) (Figure 1.2).

The Hearing Function of the Inner Ear

The human cochlea can detect sounds from 20 to 20,000 Hz.[1] Age-related hearing loss (presbycusis) typically presents with high-frequency hearing loss and varies in severity, rate of progression, and age of onset.[2,3] Noise exposure, toxic chemical exposure (ototoxicity), genetic disorders, infections, trauma, and inflammatory or autoimmune conditions are other causes of hearing loss.

Cochlea

The cochlea is a spiral-shaped structure that converts incoming sound waves into neural impulses through an auditory transduction process. The cochlea typically has about 2 1/2 turns and is about 35 mm in length.[4] The cochlea is divided into three chambers: the scala tympani, the scala media, and the scala vestibuli. The scala vestibuli and scala tympani contain perilymph, which is high in sodium. The scala media is filled with endolymph, which is more like intracellular fluid and is rich in potassium. This difference in fluid electrolyte composition is responsible for creating the endocochlear potential. The stria vascularis maintains the endocochlear potential and is located on the lateral wall of the scala media, which transports potassium into the scala media. This exchange of sodium and potassium creates an endocochlear potential in the scala media, promoting organ of Corti function.[5]

Sound Travels Through the Cochlea

The transmission of sound to the cochlea follows a series of events. First sound waves cause vibration of the tympanic membrane and the three ossicles (malleus, incus, and stapes), which causes movement of the stapes footplate against the oval window creating a fluid wave within the cochlea. The difference in surface area between the tympanic membrane and stapes footplate is about 17:1, which results in a 27 dB gain in hearing.[6] The stapes bone rocks back and forth, causing a fluid wave in the scala vestibuli. This fluid wave travels through the cochlea to the helicotrema found at the cochlea's apex. The scala vestibuli and scala tympani communicate at the helicotrema, causing the fluid wave to move down the scala tympani. The round window is located at the proximal end of the scala tympani. The round window acts as a relief valve for the fluid wave. Without the round window, the fluid would not be able to propagate through the cochlea since fluids are non-compressible.

The cochlea is arranged in a manner to have exquisite frequency selectivity. High-frequency responsive hair cells are located at the inferior basal turn, adjacent to the round window. Low- and mid-frequency sounds

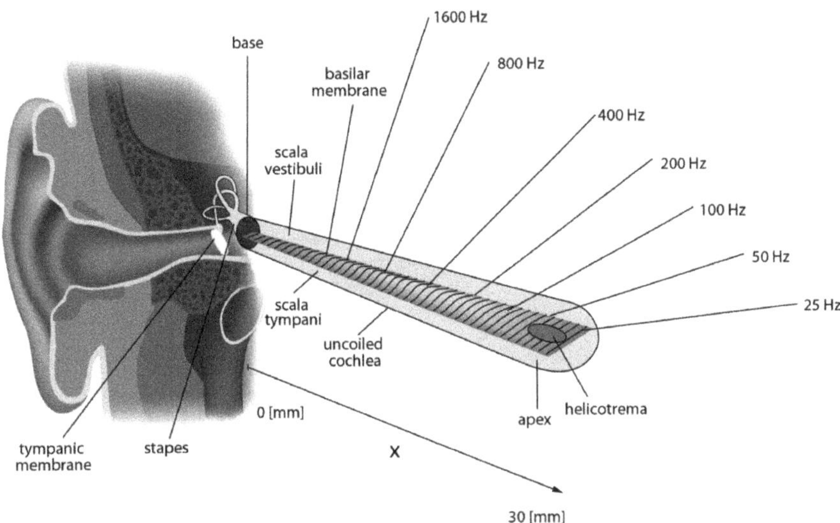

Fig. 1.3 Uncoiled cochlea highlighting tonotopic organization of the basilar membrane from the base to the apex.

(**Citation:** Uncoiled cochlea with basilar membrane from Biophysical Parameters Modification Could Overcome Essential Hearing Gaps by Kern A, Heid C, Steeb W-H, Stoop N, Stoop is licensed under CC by 2.5.)

are best detected by hair cells located at the distal apical through the middle turns of the cochlea (Figure 1.3).

Scala Media

The scala media is the functional part of the cochlea. The basilar membrane separates the scala tympani from the scala media, and Reissner's membrane separates the scala vestibuli from the scala media (Figure 1.4). The organ of Corti is located on the scala media surface of the basilar membrane. The fluid wave running through the scala vestibuli and scala tympani cause the deflection of the basilar membrane that is frequency specific. Three rows of outer hair cells (OHCs) amplify the basilar membrane displacement resulting in fine-tuned sound frequency.

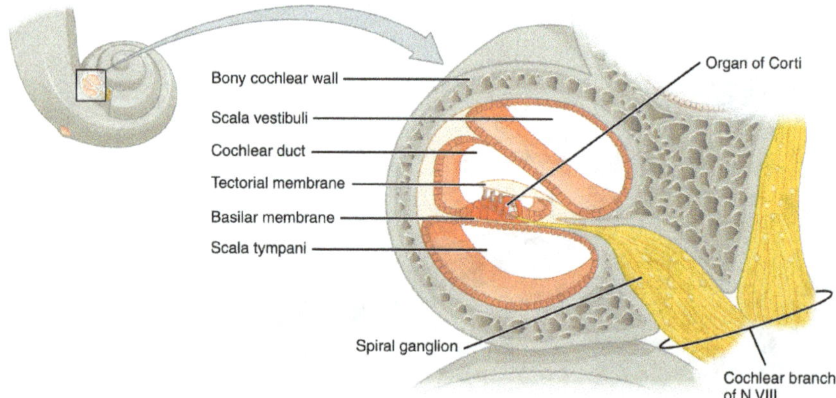

Fig. 1.4 Cross-sectional view of the cochlea showing the three cochlear chambers: scala vestibuli, scala media, and scala tympani.

(**Citation:** Cochlea from Version 8.25 from the Textbook OpenStax Anatomy and Physiology (https://cnx.org/contents/FPtK1zmh@8.25:fEI3C8Ot@10/Preface) by OpenStax is licensed under CC by 4.0.)

Modiolus

The modiolus is the central bony core of the cochlea that surrounds spiral ganglion cells. The spiral ganglion cells connect to the basal ends of inner hair cells (IHCs) and OHCs through nerve endings travelling via Rosenthal's canal. The neurons extending medially from the spiral ganglion cells traverse the cribriform area of the internal auditory canal and form the cochlear nerve.

Organ of Corti

The organ of Corti is a complex structure that includes the basilar membrane, IHCs, and OHCs, as well as numerous supporting cells. The basilar membrane attaches to the modiolus through a bony structure called the osseous spiral lamina that extends to the outer wall of the cochlea, where it attaches to the spiral ligament. The organ of Corti has one row of IHCs and three rows of OHCs. In addition, numerous

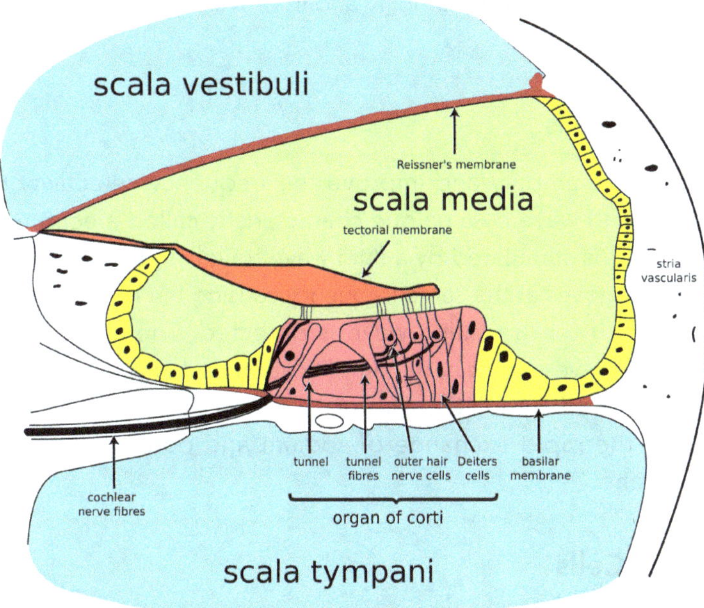

Fig. 1.5 Organ of Corti components: basilar membrane, tectorial membrane, IHCs and OHCs.

(**Citation:** Cross section of the cochlea by Oarih Ropshkow is licensed under CC by-SA 3.0.)

supporting cells within the organ of Corti work in conjunction with the hair cells and facilitate the preservation of the endocochlear potential (Figure 1.5).

Basilar Membrane

The vibration of the basilar membrane results in the activation of hair cells via the displacement of apically located stereocilia. The activated hair cells then stimulate the spiral ganglion cell's nerve endings. The stereocilia of the OHCs are embedded in the tectorial membrane, and the stereocilia of the IHCs are close enough to be displaced by the motion of the basilar membrane. The IHCs primarily detect the movement of the basilar membrane, while the OHCs amplify and improve the frequency of basilar membrane movement.

Outer Hair Cells

Outer hair cells amplify and improve the frequency selectivity of the travelling sound wave by a unique characteristic called electromotility.[7] When an OHC is stimulated by a fluid wave travelling through the cochlea, the OHC moves at the same frequency causing the basilar membrane to move only if the travelling wave is detected. The amplification of the travelling wave results in the amplification and improved frequency selectivity caused by OHCs. The OHCs can perform electromotility because of the rapid exchange of sodium and potassium across the cell membrane.

Inner Hair Cells

Inner hair cells are located closer to the modiolus than the OHCs and form one row of cells. The IHCs are the sensory receptors of the inner ear. Movement of the basilar membrane causes the stereocilia of the IHCs to bend, allowing potassium to enter the cell, which results in depolarization and stimulation of the auditory nerve.

The Vestibular Function of the Inner Ear

The vestibular portion of the inner ear is a paired, bilateral system responsible for gaze stabilization. The semicircular canals are responsible for the detection of rotational motion. At the same time, the otolith organs are responsible for detecting translational motion and determining the head's position relative to gravity. The vestibular system, like the cochlea, is surrounded by dense otic capsule bone, which is filled with perilymph, which surrounds the endolymph-filled membranous labyrinth.

Figure 1.6. Overview of the vestibular system. The three semicircular canals detect rotational motion and the utricle and saccule detect linear and

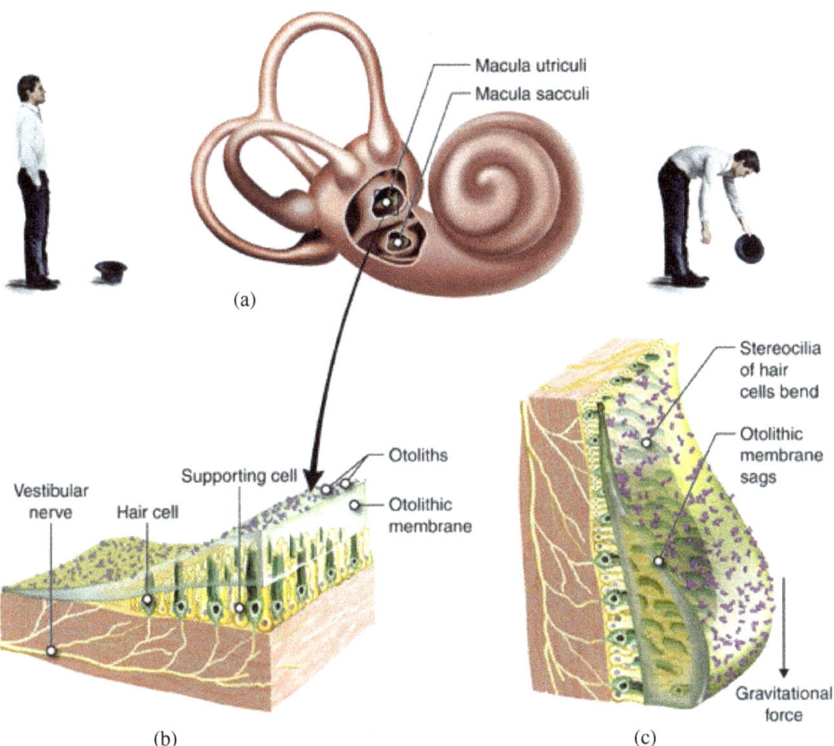

Fig. 1.6 Utricle and saccule detect linear and gravitational movement. **(a)** Utricle and saccule within the bony labyrinth. **(b, c)** Changes in linear position cause movement of the otolithic membrane triggering action potentials within the hair cells.

(**Citation:** Structure and Function of the Semicircular Canals by Cenveo is licensed under CC by-SA 3.0.)

gravitational motion. The vestibular system is stimulated by the movement of stereocilia of vestibular hair cells (Figures 1.6, 1.7).

Vestibule

The vestibule is an ovoid-shaped cavity between the lateral aspect of the internal auditory canal and the medial to the oval window. A mobile stapes footplate fills the oval window on the lateral part of the vestibule.

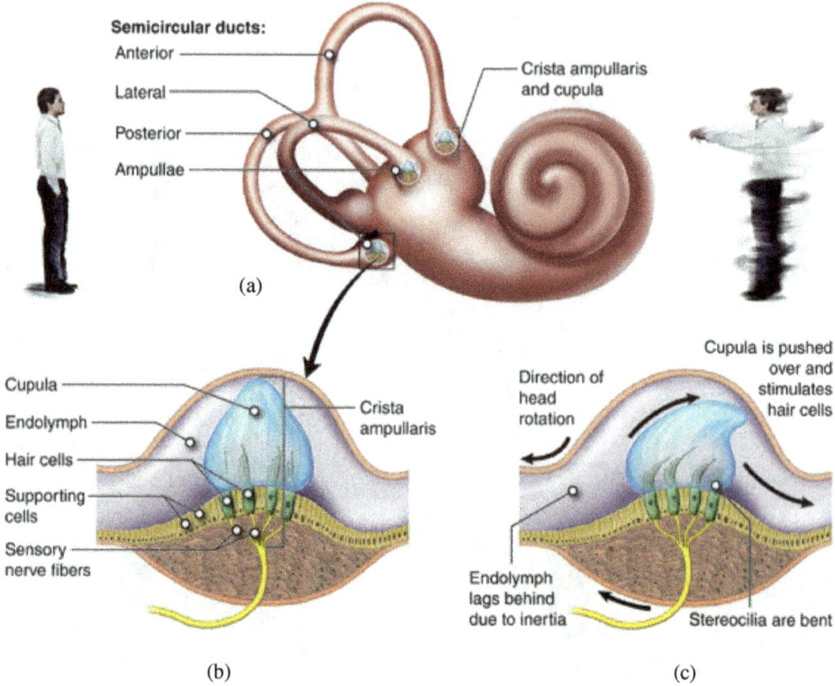

Fig. 1.7 Three semicircular canals detect rotational movement. **(a)** Each semicircular canal has a dilated end known as the ampulla, which contains the crista ampullaris and cupula. **(b, c)** Rotational movement triggers fluid wave within the endolymph causing movement of the cupula stimulating hair cells.

(**Citation:** Structure of the Maculae by Cenveo is licensed under CC by-SA 3.0.)

There are additional openings into the vestibule, including three from the ampullated ends of the superior, lateral, and posterior semicircular canals, a non-ampullated end of the lateral canal semicircular, the common crus, the ductus reunions, and the utricular-saccular duct. The utricle and saccule are the membranous otolith organs located in the elliptical and spherical recess, respectively, along the medial wall of the vestibule.

Saccule

The membranous saccule, located in the anterior medial aspect of the vestibule, is vertically oriented, which allows it to detect the head's position relative to gravity. The saccule also detects any head movement in the vertical plane. The saccular macula contains hair cells that are oriented facing away from a centrally located ridge called the striola. A thick gel-like substance covers the hair cells, which is maintained by supporting cells. On the surface of the gel-like substance and near the hair cells are crystal structures made of calcium carbonate, referred to as otoliths. The otoliths are denser than the surrounding endolymph and thus deflect towards gravity or in the opposite direction of movement. Movement of the otoliths and the underlying gel-membrane results in activation or inhibition of the underlying hair cells. Hair cell activation or inhibition then respectively increases or decreases the constant firing rate of the associated vestibular nerve fibers attached to the medial surface of the hair cells. The saccular nerve is a branch of the inferior vestibular nerve that terminates in the vestibular nuclei. The membranous saccule is in continuity with the cochlea via the ductus reunions. The saccule is also in continuity with the utricle and ELD via the uticulo-saccular duct.

Utricle

Compared to the saccule, the utricle is located more posterior and superior along the medial wall of the vestibule and is in continuity with the semicircular canals. The utricle is oriented horizontally and detects motion in that plane. The utricular macula also contains hair cells opposite the saccule and the cells are oriented towards the centrally located ridge known as the striola. Activation or inhibition of the utricular hair cells results in an increase or decrease in neural impulses from the utricular nerve, which is a branch of the superior vestibular nerve. The superior vestibular nerve terminates in the vestibular nuclei within the brainstem.

Semicircular Canals

The three semicircular canals are aligned at right angles and paired with a semicircular canal on the contralateral side. The lateral semicircular canals are paired, and the contralateral posterior and superior canals are paired. This redundancy allows for compensation in the event of a unilateral vestibular injury. Furthermore, each canal has a dilated end known as the ampulla. The ampulla contains the crista ampullaris, a ridge-like structure covered with hair cells. The cupula is a membranous structure that sits on the outer surface of the hair cells. A rotational movement in the plane of the semicircular canal results in stimulation or inhibition of the hair cells, depending on the direction of rotation. The hair cells then increase or decrease the firing rate of their respective vestibular nerves connected at their basal ends. The superior and lateral semicircular canal nerves are branches of the superior vestibular nerve. In contrast, the singular nerve of the inferior vestibular nerve innervates the posterior semicircular.

Endolymphatic Duct and Sac

The endolymphatic sac (ELS) is located on the dura posterior face of the petrous bone. The location of the ELS is relatively constant, but its size and osseous covering from the operculum are variable. The vestibular aqueduct, a small intraosseous channel, originates from the posterior aspect of the vestibule and extends medially to the common crus at the level of the lateral semicircular canal (Donaldson's line), where it eventually exits the posterior face of the temporal bone. The membranous ELD is 0.1–0.2 mm in diameter and originates from the saccule and utriculo-saccular duct.[8] The ELD connects to the ELS via the vestibular aqueduct.

The ELS and ELD serve several functions, including endolymph homeostasis and immunologic response within the inner ear.[9,10] The ELS/ELD has a rich vascular and lymphatic plexus. Advanced imaging techniques support the role of this system in endolymph homeostasis.[11] Inner ear-specific macrophages occur within the ELD along with lymphocytes and plasma cells, further confirming an immunologic role for this system.[12]

Conclusions

The inner ear is complex and functions as both the auditory and vestibular organ. The cochlea allows for a wide range of frequency of hearing between 20 and 20,000 Hz and the frequency-selectivity to appreciate speech and complex sounds, such as differentiating a musical instrument or listening to a symphony. The inner ear's vestibular system signals the brain to know where the body and head are in space. The remaining chapters will discuss diseases that can affect the hearing and vestibular systems.

References

1. Rossing TD. (2007) *Springer Handbook of Acoustics*. New York: Springer, xxiv, 1182 p.
2. Huang Q, Tang J. (2010) Age-related hearing loss or presbycusis. *Eur Arch Otorhinolaryngol* **267**(8):1179–91.
3. Van Eyken E, Van Camp G, Van Laer L. (2007) The complexity of age-related hearing impairment: Contributing environmental and genetic factors. *Audiol Neurootol* **12**(6):345–58.
4. Gilroy AM, MacPherson BR, Ross LM. (2008) *Atlas of Anatomy*. Stuttgart, New York: Thieme, xv, 656 p.
5. Wangemann P. (2006) Supporting sensory transduction: Cochlear fluid homeostasis and the endocochlear potential. *J Physiol* **576**(Pt 1):11–21.
6. Durrant JD, Lovrinic JH. (1984) *Bases of Hearing Science*, 2nd ed. Baltimore: Lippincott Williams & Wilkins, xxiv, 276 p.
7. Brownell WE. (1990) Outer hair cell electromotility and otoacoustic emissions. *Ear Hear* **11**(2):82–92.
8. Clarke RL, Isaacson B, Kutz JW, *et al*. (2021) MRI evaluation of the normal and abnormal endolymphatic duct in the pediatric population: A comparison with high-resolution CT. *AJNR Am J Neuroradiol* **42**(10):1865–9.
9. Bagger-Sjoback D. (1991) Modern concepts of endolymphatic sac function. *Acta Otorhinolaryngol Belg* **45**(2):165–9.
10. Lundquist PG. (1976) Aspects on endolymphatic sac morphology and function. *Arch Otorhinolaryngol* **212**(4):231–40.
11. Lo WW, Daniels DL, Chakeres DW, *et al*. (1997) The endolymphatic duct and sac. *AJNR Am J Neuroradiol* **18**(5):881–7.
12. Kampfe Nordstrom C, Danckwardt-Lilliestrom N, Laurell G, *et al*. (2018) The human endolymphatic sac and inner ear immunity: Macrophage interaction and molecular expression. *Front Immunol* **9**:3181.

2 Etiological Aspects of Hearing Loss

Maria-Pia Tuset, MD, MSc[1,2,6]; Camron Davies, MD[1,6]; Alexa Denton, MD[1,6]; Mona Roshan, MSc[1]; Jaimee N. Cooper, BS[1,6]; Adrien A. Eshraghi, MD, MSc, FACS[1,3,4,5,6]

Abstract

Hearing loss is a common disability affecting around 15% of Americans. Sensorineural hearing loss (SNHL) concerns patients presenting with inner ear or auditory nerve dysfunction. When symptoms occur, patients can feel overwhelmed and lost. This chapter aims to discuss different etiologies causing SNHL in adults and in children, as the situation is very different in both cases. Sudden SNHL will also be defined with its possible etiologies; this is a common cause of urgent care visits and requires appropriate and timely treatment or referral to an Otolaryngologist, also known as an Ear, Nose, and Throat (ENT) specialist. Diagnostic tools currently used are described, along with the differential diagnosis physicians must rule out before confirming a sensorineural disease. Treatment options and current guidelines are presented, to prepare and inform patients on the different options.

Corresponding Author: Adrien A. Eshraghi, MD, MSc, FACS

[1] Department of Otolaryngology, Hearing Research and Cochlear Implant Laboratory, University of Miami Miller School of Medicine, Miami, FL, United States

[2] Department of Otolaryngology–Head and Neck Surgery, Fondation Adolphe de Rothschild, Paris, France

[3] Department of Neurological Surgery, University of Miami Miller School of Medicine, Miami, FL, United States

[4] Department of Biomedical Engineering, University of Miami, Coral Gables, FL, United States

[5] Department of Pediatrics, University of Miami Miller School of Medicine, Miami, FL, United States

[6] Hearing Research and Cochlear Implant Laboratory of Dr. Adrien A Eshraghi, University of Miami, Miami, FL, United States

Hearing Loss in the World

Hearing loss is currently considered as one of the most prevalent chronic conditions in the United States and the third leading cause of disability worldwide. Globally, over 1.5 billion people live with hearing loss, and this number has been estimated to rise to 2.5 million in the next 25 years. In the United States, over 30 million adults, which is 15% of all Americans, have some degree of hearing loss.[1] Over 80% of patients affected by hearing loss suffer from sensorineural hearing loss (SNHL). Age-related hearing loss, also known as presbycusis, is the leading cause of SNHL. Fifty percent of adults in their 70s and 80% of those 85 years and older present with some degree of hearing loss. Despite this high prevalence, hearing loss remains undetected and thus, untreated in most of the population. Only about one-third of people with self-reported hearing loss have ever had their hearing tested. Hearing rehabilitation is essential in managing this. Conventional hearing aids are continually developed to offer better quality of sound and more discreet devices. However, only 15% of people eligible for hearing aids consistently use them, citing factors such as cost, discomfort, and social stigma. The impact is major, particularly on mental health, education, employment, and social interactions. The financial burden rises to almost a trillion dollars globally on a yearly basis. In the United States, medical costs resulting from hearing impairment range from 3.3 to 12.8 million dollars annually. This estimation includes direct medical costs, disability expenditures, and indirect costs from productivity losses and caregiver expenses.[1]

Difficulty hearing speech adversely affects social engagement and relationships. Hearing loss is associated with decreased quality of life, dementia, depression, falls, and mortality. Recent studies have shown that early detection and treatment of hearing impairment delays the onset of dementia. In hearing-impaired children,[2] delayed language development, social isolation, and academic failure are common. All of this makes management of hearing loss a worldwide priority. Communication between physicians and patients must improve for this aim. A recent survey found that in the United States, only 20.6% of patients who saw a physician in the last 5 years for a hearing complaint were referred to an otolaryngologist or audiologist for advanced hearing care. Less than 15% of physicians performed hearing tests in their offices to these patients. Approximately 80% of family care physicians were unaware that cochlear implants were covered by all health plans and 26% did not know that cochlear implants could restore hearing. This lack of information among physicians explains the high rate of cochlear implant underutilization in the United States, which is estimated to be 5% of the eligible adult population.[1]

Definition of Sensorineural Hearing Loss

Hearing loss is the partial or total inability to hear. Within this broad definition, there are numerous subtypes and descriptors that classify an individual's type and severity of hearing loss.

The first step in diagnosing hearing loss is typically done by an audiologist who assesses the intensity at which a patient begins to hear a sound. According to the World Health Organization, hearing loss is defined as the inability to hear as clearly as a person with normal hearing. In audiometry, this refers to hearing thresholds under 20 dB in both ears. However in the United States, the normal hearing threshold is usually defined by 25 dB or above (in adult). After auditory testing, hearing loss is classified as slight, mild, moderate, moderately severe, severe, or profound (Table 2.1).

For context, 20 dB is about the sound of a watch ticking, 30 dB is that of a whisper or a quiet library, and 50 dB is that of a typical conversation or moderate rainfall. Additionally, it is important to note that the dB scale is logarithmic, meaning that as the dB increases, the intensity of sounds exponentially increases so that a sound at 10 decibels is 10 times more

Table 2.1 Degree of hearing loss according to pure-tone audiometry hearing thresholds.

Severity	Threshold (in dB)
Slight (children)	16–25 (children)
Mild	26–40
Moderate	41–55
Moderately severe	56–70
Severe	71–90
Profound	>90

intense than a sound at 1 dB. In contrast, a sound at 100 dB is one billion times more intense than a sound at 10 dB. Furthermore, when discussing dB, 'sound intensity' and 'loudness' are not synonyms. Intensity represents the scientific measure of a sound wave's power, whereas loudness describes one's perception of a sound. For example, a sound perceived as loud in a quiet room may not be as loud on a busy street. However, a general rule of thumb is that for every 10 dB increase in intensity, a sound is perceived as twice as loud.

After the level of hearing loss is established, it is further characterized as either conductive, sensorineural, or mixed hearing loss. Briefly, conductive hearing loss is caused by the inability of sound to be transmitted across the outer and middle ear to the inner ear. Normally, the inner ear is the end recipient of the sound waves and converts their physical vibrations into an electrical stimulus that the brain can eventually understand. Conversely, SNHL, which will be expanded upon later in this chapter, is the inability of the inner ear or auditory nerve to transmit its electrical signal to the brain. Mixed hearing loss includes both conductive and sensorineural components (Table 2.2.).

Additionally, several other terms describe an individual's hearing loss. 'Unilateral' or 'bilateral' describes whether the deficiency is in one or both ears, respectively. 'Symmetrical' or 'asymmetrical' hearing loss is when

Table 2.2 Components of the external, middle, and inner ear.

External ear
Pinna, or auricle, refers to the outer visible portion of the ear
External ear canal
Tympanic membrane (eardrum): separates the external ear from the middle ear
Middle ear (tympanic cavity)
Ossicular chain problem (malleus, incus, stapes)
Ossicular ligaments and tendons
Middle ear cavity bone
Eustachian tubes
Inner ear
Cochlea
Vestibule (utricle, saccule), semi-circular canals

the level of impairment is the same or different in both ears. 'Progressive' or 'sudden' characterizes the onset of hearing loss as gradual or sudden. Lastly, 'congenital' or 'acquired/delayed' demonstrates whether the hearing loss was present at birth or developed later in life.

This chapter focuses on SNHL, which we will now discuss in more detail. As mentioned earlier, SNHL occurs due to the inability of the inner ear (i.e., the cochlea) to convert the mechanical energy of sound waves into electrical energy or the inability of the auditory nerve to transmit this signal to the brain. In general, this can occur through several mechanisms that damage the cochlea or the auditory nerve. For example, noise trauma can damage the cochlea's sensory cells, thereby preventing mechanical to electrical transduction. Also, atypical fetal development can result in the failure to produce a functional auditory nerve that transmits the electrical impulse from the cochlea to the brain. Overall, SNHL has several known causes that result in various pathophysiologies, treatments, and prognoses. We will continue to discuss these etiologies in the next section.

Etiologies of Sensorineural Hearing Loss

Etiologies in Adults

Sensorineural hearing loss is caused by many factors, which include genetics, aging, and/or external factors. Some causes remain unknown amongst the medical community. The common causes that affect adults include age-related hearing loss, drug-induced hearing loss, noise-induced hearing loss (NIHL), otosclerosis, Meniere's diseases, temporal bone fractures, infections, neoplasms, autoimmune hearing loss, chronic otitis, and sudden SNHL.

Age-related hearing loss

Age-related hearing loss, which is also known as presbycusis, is the most common cause of acquired hearing loss. Although individuals can start experiencing loss of high-frequency sounds in their mid-50s and 60s, age-related hearing loss affects nearly two-thirds of those who are 70-years old. Most of the available research shows that the cause is related to damage to different structures within the inner ear, especially the hair cells. Besides the aging process itself, there are many known factors that are correlated with this damage; however, the exact cause is not completely understood. Some studies show that there are correlations with genetic factors, alcohol and cigarette use, and high blood pressure; however, more research is needed. Due to the aging population in the United States, the burden of this condition has increased, which also affects the quality of life of elderly individuals. Older patients who have significant hearing loss are at higher risk of depression, falls, isolation, loneliness, and dementia.[3]

Drug-induced hearing loss

There are medications on the market that are known to be toxic to the inner ear. These include some specific chemotherapy drugs and antibiotics, among others. Although some of these medications are used sparingly or even avoided due to their side effect profile, others may be needed if there are no alternatives. One example is **cisplatin**, which is a chemotherapeutic agent used in the treatment of solid malignancies. Despite its benefit in fighting cancer, it produces damaging free radicals that are toxic to the inner ear structures, leading to hearing loss. When a patient has hearing loss from cisplatin, they can experience various ranges of auditory dysfunction that affect one or both ears. The effect of cisplatin on the inner ear is dependent on the amount of the drug used, the patient's age, if the patient is also receiving radiotherapy, and other pretreatment factors. Around half of patients who undergo chemotherapy treatment with greater than 200 mg doses of cisplatin will experience a noticeable reduction in hearing in both ears.[4]

Similarly, there are various classes of antibiotics that affect the functioning of the inner ear. The most commonly discussed are **aminoglycosides**, such as amikacin, kanamycin, gentamicin, and tobramycin, which are used to treat many different types of infections. It is thought that the generation of harmful byproducts, like the mechanism of cisplatin, results in potentially irreversible damage. The range of hearing loss depends specifically on the medication used, dosage, and length of treatment. It is estimated that roughly 20–50% of patients treated with oral aminoglycosides may experience hearing loss.

Other medications that are known to cause hearing loss are **non-steroidal anti-inflammatory drugs (NSAIDs)**, such as ibuprofen and acetaminophen. These medications, which are amongst the most common over-the-counter drugs taken for pain and inflammation, can also decrease blood flow to the cochlea and ultimately lead to hearing loss. **Loop diuretics**, which are commonly used to treat high blood pressure, heart failure, and fluid overload, are another class of medications that can be associated with hearing loss. These medications affect the transport of certain ions that are responsible for regulating the fluid in the inner ear, the component involved in sending auditory signals to the brain. There are many other medications that are linked to hearing loss and will be listed further in Table 2.3.

Noise-induced hearing loss

Noise-induced hearing loss is caused by overexposure to loud noises or acoustic trauma, which can lead to loss or damage of sensory hair cells responsible for sending sound signals to the brain. The inner ear hair cells make connections, known as synapses, with nerve fibers that send auditory signals to the brain. Studies have shown that noise can also permanently damage these synapses, and ultimately lead to hearing loss.[5] This damage is termed synaptopathies and is an emerging area of research. According to the CDC, nearly 40 million adults in the United States have experienced some degree of NIHL, and in 2015, the World Health Organization claimed that 1.1 billion teenagers and young adults aged 12–35 are at risk of NIHL from exposure to loud sounds without adequate hearing protection (United States Department of Health and Human Services). NIHL is common in individuals who attend loud events or use firearms frequently. As society becomes more industrialized, the number of individuals exposed to acoustic trauma is suspected to increase.

Sudden sensorineural hearing loss

Sudden sensorineural hearing loss (SSNHL) is the loss of at least 30 dB of hearing in 3 or more frequencies in no more than 3 days. In the United States, anywhere between 5 and 30 cases per 100,000 people have reported some degree of SSNHL, and these statistics closely reflect those of other countries.[6] SSNHL usually occurs in one ear; however, approximately 1–2% of patients experience loss in both ears. Unfortunately, the damage that leads to SSNHL is usually permanent, with the underlying cause unknown in about 85–90% of cases.[7] Some known causes include viral infections and autoimmune conditions, but in most cases, the cause remains unknown. When the etiology

Table 2.3 Ototoxic drugs that may cause hearing loss.

Drug category	Drug class	Drug subclass	Drug names
Antimicrobials	Antibiotics	– Aminoglycosides (+++)	– Tobramycin, netilmicin, amikacin, neomycin, kanamycin, streptomycin, gentamicin
		– Macrolides	– Clarithromycin, azithromycin, erythromycin, roxithromycin
		– Tetracycline	– Doxycycline, minocycline
		– Quinolones	– Ciprofloxacin, ofloxacin, norfloxacin, moxifloxacin
		– Other	– Vancomycin, chloramphenicol, trimethoprim-sulfamethoxazole, imipenem, sulfadiazine, metronidazole, polymyxin B and E
	Antivirals	– Anti-herpetic (herpes)	– Ganciclovir, valganciclovir
		– Anti-retroviral (HIV)	– Zalcitabine
		– Interferons	– Ribavirin + interferon
	Antifungals		– Amphotericin B
	Antimalarial		– Quinine, hydroxychloroquine, primaquine, quinidine
Analgesics	Anti-inflammatory and acetaminophen	– Nonsteroidal anti-inflammatory drugs (NSAIDs)	– Ibuprofen, diclofenac, naproxen, celecoxib, ketoprofen
		– Salicylates	– Aspirin, choline salicylate, sulfasalazine
			– Acetaminophen
	Opiates		– Buprenorphine, oxycodone, tramadol, naltrexone

Cytotoxic and immuno-suppressive drugs	Cytotoxic drugs	– Platinum compounds (+++)	– Cisplatin, carboplatin
		– Vinca alkaloids	– Vindesine, vincristine
		– Other	– Paclitaxel, cyclophosphamide, ifosfamide, bleomycin
	Immunosuppressive drugs		– Cyclosporine, mycophenolate, tacrolimus, methotrexate
Cardiovascular drugs	Antihypertensives	– Loop diuretics (++)	– Furosemide, ethacrynic acid, bumetanide
		– Thiazides	– Hydrochlorothiazide, indapamide
		– Potassium sparing diuretics	– Amiloride, eplerenone
		– Carbonic anhydrase inhibitors	– Acetazolamide
		– ACE inhibitor	– Enalapril, ramipril
		– Angiotensin II inhibitor antagonist	– Irbesartan, losartan, telmisartan, valsartan, olmesartan
		– Calcium channel blockers	– Nicardipine, amlodipine, nimodipine, nifedipine
	Antiarrhythmics and rate controlling drugs	– Beta blockers	– Metoprolol, atenolol, carvedilol
		– Calcium channel blockers	– Diltiazem, verapamil
		– Others	– Flecainide
	Lipid lowering drugs	– Statin	– Atorvastatin
Neurologic drugs		– Anticonvulsant	– Sodium valproate
		– Anti-Parkinson's disease	– Entacapone

is unknown, the term 'idiopathic sensorineural hearing loss' is used. There will be further discussion on SSNHL throughout the remaining chapters.

Meniere's disease

Individuals diagnosed with Meniere's disease have a triad of symptoms that include hearing loss, vertigo, and tinnitus. Although the exact cause of Meniere's disease is not fully understood, one theory is that it is caused by an excess of fluid in the inner ear (hydrops) that is responsible for helping with transmission of sound. Some theories on the pathophysiology of Meniere's include immune disorders, electrolyte imbalance of the inner ear, allergies, and migraine. Definite Meniere's is defined as two or more episodes of vertigo that last from 20 minutes to 12 hours, low to mid-frequency SNHL in at least one ear before, during, or after 1 vertigo episode, and tinnitus and/or fullness in the affected ear. Probable Meniere's is defined as two or more episodes of vertigo or dizziness, lasting 20 minutes to 24 hours, fluctuating aural symptoms (tinnitus, fullness) and symptoms not explained better by another vestibular diagnosis that may lead to SNHL, tinnitus, and vertigo must be ruled out before a definitive diagnosis can be made.

Otosclerosis

Otosclerosis results from abnormal bone remodeling within the ear that leads to ossicular chain blockage and ultimately hearing loss. Although otosclerosis usually leads to conductive hearing loss when the bones of the middle ear are affected, SNHL occurs when otosclerotic foci develop in the otic capsule and the surrounding inner ear structures. Although the cause of otosclerosis in patients is usually unknown, some degree of a genetic component is thought to contribute to developing otosclerosis, with 60% of patients reporting a family history of the condition.[8] Caucasians are at a significantly higher risk, and it is also more common in women. Some studies have proposed an association with some viral illnesses, such as measles.[9] Although the abnormal bone remodeling usually starts in patients in their 20s or 30s, patients will not start to experience its effects until they are in their 40s. This can occur in one or both ears. Because of the progressive nature of this condition, patients will experience early symptoms of conductive hearing loss, such as loss of low-frequency sounds. However, as the condition progresses or impacts the cochlea, patients can develop mixed hearing loss. Because this condition usually affects the middle ear ossicles, SNHL is rare, occurring in about 10% of cases.[10]

Temporal bone fractures

The temporal bone is adjacent to the ear on each side of the skull and houses its associated structures. Since the middle and inner ear structures are very fragile, any direct mechanical disruption can lead to hearing loss. Although the inner ear structures are well protected inside the dense otic capsule of the temporal bone, fractures may occur as in any other bones in the body. When this is the case, SNHL will occur. The temporal bone itself is made up of four different bones: the mastoid process, the tympanic portion, the squamosa, and the petrous apex. Damage to any of these structures will dictate the specific symptoms the patient will experience in relation to their hearing. Imaging is recommended in cases of trauma to evaluate damage caused to the middle and inner ear. However, it is sometimes difficult to visualize microfractures in the region attributed to SNHL. Hearing evaluation should always be performed on patients with temporal bone trauma once they are stable enough.

Infectious causes

There are various infections that affect the ear which are associated with hearing loss. The most common and well known is otitis media, which is an infection of the middle ear by bacteria or fungi. The inflammation associated with an acute infection can lead to a conductive hearing loss since it can affect the functioning of the tympanic membrane and ossicles. However, in chronic otitis media, the toxins generated from the infection can leak into the fluid of the inner ear, and ultimately lead to irreversible damage to the cochlea. Even though this association has been studied, it is not known how long the chronic infection or how many otitis media infections must occur to lead to SNHL.[11]

Viral infections are also known to cause various degrees of SNHL. Some common viruses known to infect the ear in different ways include herpes simplex virus, HIV, hepatitis viruses, measles, mumps, rubella, and cytomegalovirus. There are some theories described in the literature that suggest that viruses can lead to hearing loss, whether it is by a new infection or the reactivation of a virus that stays dormant after the first infection. One theory includes direct infection of the nerve responsible for transmitting sounds known as the cochlear nerve. This infection is known as neuritis and ranges in severity and time of infection. Another theory is infection of the fluid and soft tissues of the cochlea structures. This is called labyrinthitis, which can also include symptoms of hearing loss and vertigo-like symptoms. Lastly, a more complicated theory includes a virus that is infecting another region in the body. The antibodies made to fight that virus cross-react with the structures of the inner ear causing an inflammatory response that can lead to hearing loss. Finally, the specific case of a particular infection, meningitis, needs to be discussed. Meningitis refers to infection of the meninges, the protective layers surrounding the brain. In this case, infectious agents spread through the cerebrospinal fluid that is connected to the inner ear fluids, also leading to hearing loss in some cases. Audiometry testing is therefore recommended in cases of meningitis.

Neoplastic causes

When a patient presents with one-sided or asymmetrical hearing loss, it is important to consider neoplastic causes of hearing loss, which include both malignant and benign tumors. The most common neoplastic cause of hearing loss is a vestibular schwannoma, also known as an acoustic neuroma. These tumors are benign growths that arise from the vestibular nerve and can lead to hearing loss and tinnitus. They can be diagnosed by magnetic resonance imaging (MRI) studies. The yearly incidence of this tumor is about 10.4 per million. Although a majority occur unilaterally, they can occur bilaterally in about 5% of cases, which is usually associated with a genetic condition known as neurofibromatosis type II. Although rare, another tumor that can lead to SNHL is an endolymphatic sac tumor. The endolymphatic sac is a structure that is associated with the endolymph fluid of the inner ear and has a role in monitoring its pressure and volume. The tumor that arises from this structure can be both sporadic or associated with Von Hippel-Lindau disease, a condition that will present in patients as progressive hearing loss. Other symptoms can include tinnitus, vertigo, ear pain, and difficulty moving the face, depending on the extent of growth of the tumor. Although the tumor is usually slow growing and rarely metastases, it can be locally destructive. MRI with and without gadolinium contrast should be considered in patients with these symptoms without a known cause.

Autoimmune hearing loss

One of the rarest causes of hearing loss includes autoimmune hearing loss. This type of SNHL accounts for about <1% of hearing loss in patients. Despite this low number, it is a current area of research due to the severe impact it has on patients. It commonly affects women in their 40s to 60s.[12] Autoimmune hearing loss can be separated into both primary and secondary causes. Primary autoimmune hearing loss results from a condition that only affects the inner ear. Secondary autoimmune hearing loss occurs when the patient's preexisting autoimmune condition affects the ears. Although the mechanism for autoimmune hearing loss is currently unclear, there are two hypotheses for how it may occur. The first is that autoantibodies and immune cells, namely T-cells, attack the body itself, including parts of the inner ear. In this hypothesis, an innate or foreign antigen initiates the adaptive immune system, these cells are then able to penetrate the blood-labyrinthine barrier and reach the inner ear. The second is that antibody complexes depositing in blood vessels cause inflammation in the inner ear. The presence of these antibodies and/or immune cells can cause obstruction of the small blood vessels of the inner ear causing ischemia and release of cytokines or formation of the inflammasome and activation of programmed cell death. Because autoimmune hearing loss has many different causes, there is no reliable diagnostic test for the condition. Diagnosis is made by the patient's history, ruling out other causes of hearing loss, and the patient's response to therapies such as corticosteroids and/or immunosuppressants. Patients will usually present with progressive hearing loss in either one or both ears over the span of months. If the patient's hearing loss responds to corticosteroids or immunosuppressants, blood testing is recommended to evaluate for other markers of autoimmune conditions.

Etiologies in Children

Congenital hearing loss

Congenital hearing loss, or hearing loss present at birth, can be a result of many factors in utero and occurs in about 1.1 per 1,000 newborns. The most common causes of congenital SNHL are related to genetic mutations of a single gene that are either passed down to the fetus or occur spontaneously. Many of these genetic conditions, such as Jervell and Lange-Nielsen disease, affect various structures of the middle ear and inner ear, leading to abnormalities in sound transmitted to the brain.[2] Although a single gene is most commonly the culprit for genetic hearing loss in a neonate, other genetic causes of hearing loss are due to well-known syndromes that lead to abnormalities throughout the body. Additionally, some infections such as cytomegalovirus and rubella virus that occur in utero are known to cause an acquired SNHL. Hearing loss in a newborn can be detected early on, usually within the first few months of birth with appropriate screening (using acoustic emissions testing or ABRs). When an abnormality in the screening test is found, it is important to identify the cause so that proper interventions can be taken to prevent speech and language delay.

Genetic causes of hearing loss

Genetic factors account for over 50% of congenital hearing loss (Figure 2.1). In around 20–25% of cases, the hearing loss occurs in conjunction with a constellation of other symptoms due to an underlying genetic abnormality; these are termed syndromes. In the other 75–80% of cases, hearing loss

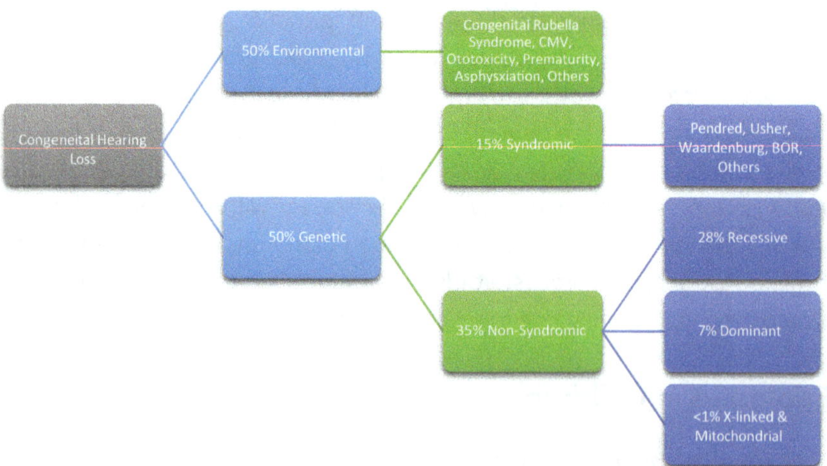

Figure 2.1 Causes of congenital hearing loss, as described by Smith *et al.*[13]

is isolated and is conversely termed non-syndromic hearing loss. In addition to these subgroups, there are several different inheritance patterns for SNHL, and most of the time, both parents have normal hearing, which makes understanding these genetic causes particularly important.

Non-syndromic hearing loss

Non-syndromic hearing loss can be further divided into two inheritance types: autosomal recessive and autosomal dominant. In autosomal dominant non-syndromic hearing loss, typically at least one parent or grandparent of the child has the same type of hearing loss, and there is at least a 50% probability of passing on the gene to a child. In these cases, there is usually the expectation that a child will be affected since the parents have been affected. In contrast, for autosomal recessive hearing loss, typically both parents have a single copy of the gene causing hearing loss, but in their cases, the phenotype of the gene is suppressed by another functional copy of the gene. Consequently, and most concerning for parents, children with this type of hearing loss are born to parents with normal hearing. Genetically, since both parents have one copy of the functional gene and one copy of the hearing loss gene, there is a 25% chance of their child having hearing loss. There are over 100 genes known to cause non-syndromic hearing loss, including GJB2, MYO15A, and STRC.[2] Mutations in this gene cause abnormalities to ion transportation within the inner ear, impairing the ability to convert mechanical sound waves into electrical signals that the brain can process.

Syndromic hearing loss

As mentioned previously, ~15% of congenital hearing loss are part of syndromes. A syndrome is a set of symptoms that occur together and suggest the presence of a certain disease or an increased chance of developing the disease. A few of the most common hereditary syndromes associated with hearing loss are Pendred syndrome, Usher syndrome, Alport syndrome, branchio-oto-renal (BOR) syndrome, and CHARGE syndrome.

Pendred syndrome is characterized by severe to profound sensorineural hearing impairment, balance dysfunction, and thyroid issues.

Waardenburg syndrome is another common cause of syndromic hearing loss. It is characterized by altered pigmentation of the skin, eyes, and hair, in addition to hearing loss.

Usher syndrome has three subtypes, which variably affect both hearing and vision. Types I and II are the most common subtypes, while type III is much less common.[14] Type I presents with profound hearing loss or complete deafness at birth, balance problems, and loss of vision beginning around age 10. Type II presents with severe hearing loss beginning in early childhood with loss of vision starting as a teenager yet normal balance. Type III presents with normal hearing at birth that becomes progressive hearing loss starting in early childhood, loss of vision during the teenage years, and normal balance. Early intervention and treatment may help manage some symptoms. Extensive research is being conducted in this area.

Alport syndrome is characterized by progressive SNHL beginning in late childhood, blood in the urine progressing to kidney failure, and vision problems. Notably, these symptoms are usually worse in males than in females.

Branchio-oto-renal syndrome generally presents at birth with embryonically-related abnormalities, including fistulas (i.e., passages connecting the throat to the surface of the neck), neck cysts, malformations of the outer, middle, and inner ear, hearing loss, and kidney problems.

CHARGE syndrome, an acronym for its major symptoms (coloboma, heart defects, atresia of choanae, retardation of growth, genital abnormalities, and ear abnormalities), also presents at birth with ear abnormalities, which include mild to profound hearing loss.

Inner ear malformations

Inner ear malformations (IEMs) account for roughly 20% of SNHL cases.[15] IEMs are generally due to abnormal fetal development. Importantly, the timing and severity of the inciting event has a significant effect on the development of the malformation, with earlier and larger insults leading to worse IEMs. IEMs can be classified based on the Sennaroglu criteria and their different subtypes and are summarized in Table 2.4. Major IEMs are presented in Figure 2.2. It is important to note that while hearing loss due to IEMs can be restored via cochlear implantation, there is an increased

Table 2.4 Inner ear malformations.

IEM	Description	Audiological findings
Common cavity deformity	Vestibule and cochlea are combined into one round structure.	Profound sensorineural hearing loss
Michel deformity	Absence of cochlea, vestibule, semicircular canals, vestibular and cochlear aqueducts.	Profound sensorineural hearing loss
Cochlear aplasia	Absence of a cochlea. Multiple forms with normal labyrinth or dilated vestibule.	Profound sensorineural hearing loss
Hypoplastic cochlea	Cochlea and vestibule are clearly separated but cochlea's external dimensions are smaller than normal.	Partial sensorineural, conductive, or mixed hearing loss
Enlarged vestibular aqueduct syndrome	Normal cochlea, vestibule, and semicircular canals with a vestibular aqueduct that is larger than 1.5 mm.	Spectrum of normal hearing to profound mixed or sensorineural hearing loss that may be progressive in nature
Incomplete partition type I	Cochlea and vestibule are clearly separated but lacks the modiolus and interscalar septa.	Profound sensorineural hearing loss
Incomplete partition type II	Cochlea and vestibule are clearly separated, but the apical portion of modiolus is malformed.	Spectrum of normal hearing to profound mixed or sensorineural hearing loss that may be progressive in nature
Incomplete partition type III	The internal acoustic meatus is wide and is directly opened onto the basal turn of the cochlea.	Mixed or sensorineural hearing loss

risk of complications since the underlying anatomy of the inner ear has been significantly altered.[16] This requires appropriate imaging evaluation and an experienced cochlear implant surgeon.

Infection-related hearing loss

Congenital infections can lead to congenital hearing loss. For approximately half of children born with hearing loss, the underlying cause is a maternal infection during pregnancy. While a mother can have a variety of infections during pregnancy, only a few can cross the placenta and cause

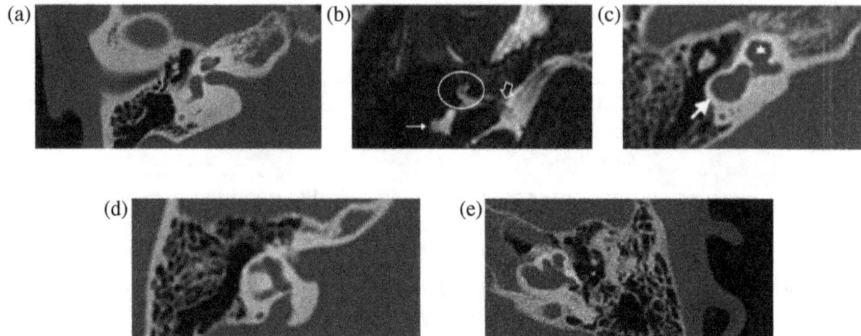

Figure 2.2 Inner ear malformations: CT temporal bone scans **(a, c–e)** and MRI **(b)** of the inner ear including **(a)** normal inner ear, **(b)** cochlear hypoplasia, **(c)** incomplete partition type I — cystic cochlea, **(d)** incomplete partition type II — Mondini malformation, and **(e)** enlarged vestibular aqueduct (EVA). Panels **(d, e)** have been taken from Feraco *et al.*[17] under the Creative Commons license.

congenital hearing loss in the fetus. Typically grouped by the mnemonic TORCHES, these are toxoplasmosis, 'others,' rubella, cytomegalovirus, herpes simplex viruses, and syphilis. As the knowledge of hearing loss and maternal infections has increased, the 'others' category has expanded to include HIV, varicella-zoster virus, rubeola, lymphocytic choriomeningitis virus (LCMV), and more. During the mid-20th century, the development of vaccines against diseases like measles dramatically reduced its impact on congenital hearing loss. However, these vaccine-preventable diseases are still common in developing countries. Currently, in the United States, congenital CMV is the most common cause of congenital hearing loss affecting approximately 1 in 200 children at birth, of which approximately 5% develop permanent hearing loss.[18]

Acquired hearing loss

Acquired hearing loss presents occasionally after birth and can be due to trauma, medication, and autoimmune disorders, as well as some of the same causes of congenital hearing loss like infection and genetics. Compared to congenital hearing loss, acquired hearing loss is much more common. In the United States, while about 2–3 children in 1,000 are born with hearing loss, by the time children are between ages 6 and 19 years of age, this number increases to about 15 in 100 (CDC data). Of the acquired causes of hearing loss, infections are the most common and include measles, mumps, Lyme disease, varicella zoster, bacterial meningitis, and occasionally, otitis media. Many of these infections like measles and mumps are preventable with vaccines, which stresses the importance of childhood vaccination. Postnatal birth complications are the second most common acquired etiology. The precise etiologies vary but predominantly include anything requiring prolonged admission to the neonatal intensive care unit, assisted ventilation, and blood transfusion therapy. The third most common cause is ototoxic drugs, including certain antibiotics like gentamicin and tobramycin, loop diuretics, and platinum-based chemotherapy. Treatments with these drugs require close monitoring to reduce the risk of injury to the inner ear. Trauma is also a cause of hearing loss in children. Notably, trauma-induced hearing loss (temporal bone fractures, concussion, noise, and blast) can cause conductive, sensorineural, or mixed hearing loss and can vary from mild to profound, depending on the structures damaged. Some auto-immune diseases, such as Cogan syndrome, can result in auto-immune reactions localized in the inner ear and result in hearing loss.

Sudden Sensorineural Hearing Loss

Epidemiology

Sudden sensorineural hearing loss (SSNHL), or sudden deafness, is a common complaint and reason for emergency consultation in otology and audiologic practices. It is defined as a purely SNHL of 30 dB or greater over at least three contiguous audiometric tested frequencies, occurring within 72 hours. It is most commonly unilateral, but a bilateral loss can occur in around 2% of patients and is often sequential. Severity can range from mild to total deafness, and prompt recognition is critical as medical interventions are usually effective in restoring hearing when given in a short time frame after the loss has occurred. Incidence of SSNHL can at first glance seem low, affecting around 5–27 cases per 100,000 people per year. However, this number may be underestimated since affected individuals who recover quickly do not present to medical care, making the true incidence close to 400 per 100,000 people.[6] This still concerns around 66,000 patients annually in the United States. Although SSNHL can occur at all ages, it is rare in children and affects mostly adults between 50 and 60 years old, of both biological sexes equally. Accompanying symptoms include tinnitus in 41–90% of patients and dizziness in 29–56% of patients, further suggesting a clear sensorineural involvement.[6]

Causes of Sudden SNHL (SSNHL)

Most patients with SSNHL have no identifiable cause for hearing loss, thus around 90% of cases are classified as 'idiopathic.' A large number of diseases can cause SSNHL, and the physician should conduct an exhaustive physical exam and anamnesis (interrogation) as overall health implications for the patient can be significant. Common identifiable causes of SSNHL are summarized in Table 2.5, but there are numerous other potential

Table 2.5 Identifiable causes of sudden sensorineural hearing loss.

Causes	Diagnoses
Auto-immune	Autoimmune ear disease, Behcet's disease, Cogan's syndrome, Susac syndrome, systemic lupus erythematosus, Sjogren's syndrome, vasculitides.
Infections	Viral infections (herpes zoster, herpes simplex, influenza, parainfluenza, mononucleosis, measles, mumps, cytomegaly, coxsackie, HIV, tick-borne encephalitis, hepatitis viruses). Bacterial infections (Lyme disease, syphilis, Rocky mountain spotted fever, mycoplasma, cryptococcus). Parasitic infections: Toxoplasmosis.
Inflammatory processes	Cholesteatoma with labyrinthine fistula, labyrinthitis (with otitis media, meningitis), encephalitis (multiple sclerosis).
Metabolic	Diabetes mellitus, hypothyroidism.
Otologic	Hydropic ear disease (Meniere's disease), otosclerosis, inner ear malformation (large vestibular aqueduct syndrome, large vestibular endolymphatic duct and sac).
Toxic	Aminoglycosides, chemotherapeutic agents, non-steroidal anti-inflammatories, salicylates, furosemide diuretic.
Traumatic	Inner ear concussion, iatrogenic trauma/surgery, perilymphatic fistula, temporal bone fracture.
Tumoral	Vestibular schwannoma, endolymphatic sac tumors, other cerebellopontine angle (CPA) tumors (meningioma, epidermoids, lipomas, facial nerve schwannoma, and metastases)
Vascular	Cerebrovascular accidents, transient ischemic attack, cerebellar infarction, inner ear hemorrhage.

differential diagnoses. Most frequent causes are infectious in 13% of cases, otologic in 5% of cases, traumatic in 4% of cases, vascular or hematologic in 3% of cases, and tumoral in 2% of cases.[6]

Many studies have proposed an association between *viral infections* and SSNHL. Herpes simplex virus or zoster (chickenpox) have shown to affect the inner ear, but clear signs of causality are difficult to obtain. One virus that has clearly shown to cause SSNHL is mumps. Concerning bacterial infections, the two most common bacteria known to cause sudden deafness are the spirochete *Borrelia burgdorferi* (Lyme disease) and *Treponema pallidum* (syphilis).

An important and relatively frequent cause of SSNHL is *vestibular schwannoma*, also referred to as acoustic neuroma. These are benign, and usually slow growing tumors developing from Schwann cells, which wrap around the nerves. Incidence is estimated to be 4%.[19] Intralabyrinthine schwannomas are in the inner ear and are rarer than vestibular schwannomas, but their incidence is probably underestimated due to their small size at time of first occurrence, or an inappropriate MRI technique for diagnosis (thick slices, brain MRI instead of temporal bone).

Vascular and hematologic diseases have often been associated with SSNHL, such as ischemic or hemorrhagic cerebrovascular attacks, transient ischemic attacks, sickle cell disease, among others. The main hypothesis is that by reducing intracochlear blood and oxygen supply to the cochlea, a transient or permanent hearing loss can be induced. The anterior inferior cerebellar artery (AICA) gives rise to the labyrinthine artery, which supplies the inner ear. Occlusion of the AICA from arteriosclerosis, immune complex deposition, inflammation, thrombosis, or vascular dissection, can lead to labyrinthine artery occlusions and cause unilateral or bilateral sudden hearing loss, tinnitus, and vestibular symptoms (dizziness, nystagmus). The labyrinthine artery gives rise to the anterior vestibular artery (providing blood supply to the utricle, superior and lateral ampullas), and the cochleovestibular artery (providing blood supply to the basal turn of the cochlea, saccule, and posterior ampulla). Cochlea vestibular artery syndrome results from vascular impairment of the cochleovestibular artery and involves isolated inner ear symptoms (sudden hearing loss and vertigo).

Finally, *hydropic ear disease* is also an important otologic cause of SNHL. With the rise of new MRI acquisition techniques, significant insight into most inner ear fluid pressure pathologies has been gained. Meniere's disease is the most known among hydropic ear diseases, with a classic triad of fluctuating SNHL, recurrent vertigo, and tinnitus. This disease is classically diagnosed during the first episode of sudden hearing loss in a patient who has experienced vertigo in the past. Endolymphatic hydrops, which refers to increased inner ear fluid pressure, can be visualized by modern MRI techniques.[20]

When the etiology of hearing loss remains unknown, patients are said to have *idiopathic sudden sensorineural hearing loss*, which is the most common cause of SSNHL to date. Several studies hypothesize on the pathophysiology of the disease. Vascular compromise, cochlear membrane rupture, and viral infection are the most accepted theories. Exhaustive testing and examination should help physicians in determining the probable cause and initiating treatment.

Treatment

When the cause of SSNHL is determined, treatment for that condition is administered. However, disease-specific therapy does not necessarily result in hearing recovery to pre-disease levels. A high rate of spontaneous resolution exists and is observed in 32–65% of patients, but physicians should not rely on this. Physicians should initiate the appropriate treatment rapidly since the window of opportunity for recovery is short.[7] Many drugs have been studied, all of which are based on the hypothesized pathophysiological mechanism of hearing loss (vascular, infectious, membrane rupture).

Steroids are the most commonly used drug prescribed for SSNHL. The inner ear expresses glucocorticoid and mineral receptors, which makes them sensitive to corticosteroid therapy. Several clinical trials have investigated the efficacy of steroid therapy, but no clear evidence of efficacy has been found for systemic (intravenous or oral) steroid treatments.[7] Oral steroids are usually a first line therapy, given the strong impact of hearing loss and tinnitus on quality of life and the mild secondary effects of short-term steroid therapy. Nonetheless, current evidence is heterogeneous with regard to systemic steroid therapy in the treatment of SSNHL. Trans-tympanic steroids can also be proposed as primary therapy, usually in combination with systemic (oral) therapy. Some use the trans-tympanic steroids treatment only as a salvage therapy when oral steroids are not helping. The main advantage of trans-tympanic therapy is that the blood–labyrinthine barrier is bypassed and higher drug concentrations can be achieved in the inner ear. Many studies on trans-tympanic therapy have shown the efficacy in recovery for patients.[7,19]

Hyperbaric oxygen therapy (HBOT) is another treatment option of SSNHL and has been considered as a potentially effective procedure. However, patients should be carefully selected (younger than 60 years old, after unsuccessful primary therapy), as there is no strong evidence on the efficacy of this treatment and the optimal patients for it.

Other therapies include antiviral, thrombolytic, vasodilators, or anti-oxidant drugs but need to be evaluated on a case-by-case basis. Complementary therapeutics were also proposed such as vitamin supplements or Ginkgo biloba but no conclusive studies on their benefits exist to date.

Prognosis

Recovery of acute SNHL will be highly dependent on the identified responsible cause. The specific disease process, duration, and treatment options for the cause will allow the physician to better inform patients on prognosis, but in most cases, hearing will not recover to previous levels. Concerning idiopathic SSNHL, as mentioned previously, a spontaneous recovery can be observed in as many as 65% of cases.[19] Several prognostic factors for hearing recovery of idiopathic SSNHL have been identified. Patients aged 60 years or older have been found to carry decreased rates of recovery along with patients with more significant hearing loss. Deafness duration of less than 2 weeks has better recovery rates while durations over 3 months have less than 10% recovery rates. Physician consultations and treatment initiation less than a week after onset present recovery rates of 87%. However, some studies suggest that the effect of early treatment may only reflect the natural history of the disease. Audiogram characteristics have also been studied. Hearing loss limited to low frequencies has the highest rate of recovery (63–88%), followed by mid-frequency losses (36–71%). There is a poor recovery rate for patients with hearing loss demonstrating a flat or down sloping audiograms and in patients with associated vertigo or imbalance.[19]

Diagnosis of Sensorineural Hearing Loss

Patients presenting with hearing loss will undergo a detailed history and physical exam from their physician. At first, the onset of hearing loss will be determined and characterized as progressive or sudden. Typical clinical features of SSNHL include a rapid decrease in hearing over 72 hours, usually noticed on awakening. The physician will evaluate for any underlying disease (cardiovascular risk, diabetes, neurological disorder, etc.), and exposure to trauma or medications. Associated symptoms such as tinnitus (sometime the main or only complaint of the patient discussed in chapter 7) and vertigo or congestive symptoms suggesting viral infection will be carefully considered. A physical examination will then be conducted. First, a diagnosis of conductive hearing loss will be excluded (ear wax blocking the outer ear canal, presence of fluids, otitis, tympanic membrane perforation), using ear microscopy and tuning fork tests. Patients with idiopathic SNHL should almost always have a normal otoscopy. Neurological disorders will be eliminated after careful examination of the cranial nerves. An exhaustive vestibular examination will be conducted, and in cases of acute vestibular syndrome, stroke will need to be excluded before any further exams are planned, using the recommended procedures.

Following patient history and physical examination, audiometry testing will need to be performed. As hearing recovery has been shown to rely on early treatment in cases of SSNHL, pure tone audiometry should be performed as soon as the diagnosis is suspected. Clinical practice guidelines recommend it within 14 days of initial examination.[7] This test allows the determination of the sensorineural nature of hearing loss as well as its severity. Treatment will be initiated at this stage by the physician. Follow-up audiometric testing will need to be performed to evaluate recovery and evaluate any further hearing degradation. Although not established as standard procedures, speech audiometry testing is highly important. Speech tests in noisy areas are more relevant regarding speech understanding, and tests in quiet areas better evaluate success of hearing aid fitting.

Auditory evoked brainstem responses (ABR) may be performed since this test studies the retrocochlear auditory pathways (sound transmission from the inner ear to the brain). This test will be able to locate whether the hearing loss stems from the cochlea or behind the cochlea (retrocochlear pathology). This exam is particularly useful in the diagnosis of vestibular schwannomas, as the presence of this tumor leads to an impairment of conduction of the auditory nerve on ABR testing.[19]

No routine labs are required when idiopathic SSNHL is suspected as there is no sufficient evidence demonstrating their benefit. Nevertheless, they can be helpful in determining the cause of hearing loss (viral infection, bacterial infection, auto-immune disease).

Patients showing neuro-otological symptoms will usually be recommended radiologic imaging. CT of temporal bones is usually not indicated in patients with SNHL, except when mixed hearing loss is observed. When an IEM is suspected, or in cases of chronic otitis, temporal bone CT is indicated. MRI with and without gadolinium contrast of the brain focusing on the internal auditory canals is gold standard.[7] Whenever possible, an MRI with hydrops protocol is preferred if hydrops is suspected. This imaging technique is emerging in many teams as the standard imaging protocols for the inner ear, as it offers better visualization of the small inner ear structures such as the saccule and the utricle, often involved in SSNHL. MRI needs to be performed to rule out vestibular schwannoma in cases of asymmetrical sensorineural hearing loss, even if hearing recovered after initial treatment. This technique is also helpful in diagnosing changes of permeability of the blood–perilymph barrier, suggesting small vascular accidents. A study found that 42% of patients with SSNHL presented MRI anomalies related to sudden deafness. No correlation between hearing loss severity and the probability of abnormal MRI was found.[20]

Differential Diagnosis of Sensorineural Hearing Loss

Most differential diagnoses of SNHL will be eliminated by the physician during anamnesis and physical examination as mentioned previously. These include mainly various causes of conductive or mixed hearing loss presented in chapter 5 of this book, such as impacted cerumen, acute otitis externa, or otitis media. In some cases, differentiating SNHL from other disorders can be difficult. We are now going to discuss in this subchapter a particular disorder long mistaken for SNHL in a wide range of patients.

Central Auditory Processing Disorders

The concept of Central auditory processing disorder (CAPD), sometimes referred to as Auditory Processing Disorder (APD), started emerging in the 1950s as auditory perception disorders not attributed to otological pathologies needed to be defined. The American Speech-Hearing-Language Association defines central auditory processing as the 'efficiency and effectiveness by which the central nervous system (CNS) utilizes auditory information as well as the perceptual processing of auditory information in the CNS and the neurobiologic activity that underlies that processing and gives rise to the electrophysiologic auditory potentials.'

From this, the term CAPD emerged and corresponds to the inability to attend to, discriminate, recognize, remember, and/or comprehend acoustic information, not related to higher-order language, cognitive, or related factors. The diagnosis is usually suspected in children by parents who report that their children have trouble hearing or understanding them. Some children will even be diagnosed with hearing loss for years before the correct diagnosis of CAPD is made.[21] Therefore, it is an important differential diagnosis of SNHL, as their ear examination will be normal. Although mostly diagnosed during childhood, CAPD can affect children and adults of all ages. Etiologies range from trauma to exposure to neurotoxic substances and neurologic disease may cause dysfunction in the central auditory nervous system, resulting in a CAPD. In addition, CAPD may coexist with and/or mimic other disorders that affect listening, learning, and communication, particularly in children.

The diagnosis of CAPD is made by specialized audiologists and can only be done after other disorders have been excluded (Autism, ADHD, hearing loss). Nevertheless, CAPD is often associated with some of these disorders. The incidence of CAPD has long been underestimated and seems to affect around 2–5% of the school-aged children, 50% of children with learning disorders, and around 75% of the elderly population.[21]

Diagnosis of CAPD requires the administration of behavioral and electrophysiologic central auditory tests. Treatment for CAPD should be individualized, deficit-specific, and multidisciplinary in nature. As research and awareness around this subject grows, patient care improves and patients strengthen their communication, learning, and listening skills, allowing for an improved quality of life.

References

1. Mahboubi H, Lin HW, Bhattacharyya N. (2018) Prevalence, characteristics, and treatment patterns of hearing difficulty in the United States. *JAMA Otolaryngol Head Neck Surg.* **144**(1):65–70.
2. Lieu JEC, Kenna M, Anne S, Davidson L. (2020) Hearing loss in children: A review. *JAMA* **324**(21):2195–205.
3. Davis A, McMahon CM, Pichora-Fuller KM, *et al.* (2016) Aging and hearing health: The life-course approach. *Gerontologist* **56**(Suppl 2):S256–67.
4. Crabb SJ, Martin K, Abab J, *et al.* (2017) COAST (cisplatin ototoxicity attenuated by aspirin trial): A phase II double-blind, randomised controlled trial to establish if aspirin reduces cisplatin induced hearing-loss. *Eur J Cancer* **87**:75–83.
5. Shi L, Chang Y, Li X, *et al.* (2016) Cochlear synaptopathy and noise-induced hidden hearing loss. *Neural Plast* **2016**:6143164.
6. Kuhn M, Heman-Ackah SE, Shaikh JA, Roehm PC. (2011) Sudden sensorineural hearing loss: A review of diagnosis, treatment, and prognosis. *Trends Amplif* **15**(3):91–105.
7. Chandrasekhar SS, Tsai Do BS, Schwartz SR, *et al.* (2019) Clinical practice guideline: Sudden hearing loss (update). *Otolaryngol Head Neck Surg* **161**(1_suppl):S1–45.
8. Babcock TA, Liu XZ. (2018) "Otosclerosis: From genetics to molecular biology." Otosclerosis and Stapes Surgery, edited by Eshraghi AA, FF Telischi, *Otolaryngol Clin North Am* **51**(2):305–18.
9. Sagar PR, Shah P, Bollampally VC, *et al.* (2020) Otosclerosis and measles: Do measles have a role in otosclerosis? A review article. *Cureus* **12**(8):e9908.
10. Quesnel AM, Ishai R, McKenna MJ. (2018) "Otosclerosis: Temporal bone pathology." Otosclerosis and Stapes Surgery, edited by Eshraghi AA, FF Telischi, *Otolaryngol Clin North Am* **51**(2):291–303.
11. Elzinga HBE, van Oorschot HD, Stegeman I, Smit AL. (2021) Relation between otitis media and sensorineural hearing loss: A systematic review. *BMJ Open* **12**(8):e050108.
12. Ribeiro R, Serôdio JF, Amaral MC, *et al.* (2021) Sensorineural hearing loss and systemic autoimmune disease: The experience of a systemic immune-mediated diseases unit. *Cureus* **13**(3):e14075.
13. Smith RJ, Bale JF Jr, White KR. (2005) Sensorineural hearing loss in children. *Lancet* **365**(9462):879–90.
14. Davies C, Bergman J, Misztal C, *et al.* (2021) The outcomes of cochlear implantation in Usher syndrome: A systematic review. *J Clin Med* **10**(13):2915.

15. Sennaroğlu L, Bajin MD. (2017) Classification and current management of inner ear malformations. *Balkan Med J* **34**(5):397–411.
16. Shah S, Walters R, Langlie J, *et al.* (2022) Systematic review of cochlear implantation in patients with inner ear malformations. *PLoS ONE* **17**(10):e0275543.
17. Feraco P, Piccinini S, Gagliardo C. (2021) Imaging of inner ear malformations: A primer for radiologists. *Radiol Med* **126**(10):1282–95.
18. Goderis J, De Leenheer E, Smets K, *et al.* (2014) Hearing loss and congenital CMV infection: A systematic review. *Pediatrics* **134**(5):972–82.
19. Plontke SK. (2017) Diagnostics and therapy of sudden hearing loss. *GMS Curr Top Otorhinolaryngol Head Neck Surg* **16**:Doc05.
20. Imai T, Uno A, Kitahara T, *et al.* (2017) Evaluation of endolymphatic hydrops using 3-T MRI after intravenous gadolinium injection. *Eur Arch Otorhinolaryngol* **274**(12):4103–11.
21. Bellis TJ, Bellis JD. (2015) Central auditory processing disorders in children and adults. *Handb Clin Neurol* **129**:537–56.

3 Prevention of Hearing Loss

Caroline Casey, BA[1]; Nina Gallo, BS[1];
Michael D. Seidman, MD, FACS[1,2,3,4]

Abstract

Hearing loss affects many individuals in the United States and has many negative impacts on both the health and quality of life of these individuals. With cases of hearing loss on the rise, there have been new technologies developed to aid in hearing; however, preventing hearing loss from the outset remains important. There are many different causes of hearing loss. With different causes such as genetic, infectious, age-related, or occupation-related, to name a few, there are different strategies that may be most effective in preventing hearing loss. Lifestyle adaptations, certain supplements, and several medications have proven to be particularly helpful in preventing hearing loss, and these changes can have a big impact not only on an individual's hearing, but also on their overall well-being.

What Causes Hearing Loss?

Over 1.5 billion people around the world suffer from hearing loss, and the World Health Organization estimates that this could rise to 2.5 billion by 2030.[1] Hearing loss greatly affects a person's ability to communicate, which impacts their overall quality of life leading to social isolation and difficulty

---

Corresponding Author: Dr. Michael D. Seidman, MD, FACS

[1] University of Central Florida College of Medicine, Orlando, FL, United States.

[2] Otology/Neurotology/Skull Base Surgery Advent Health Celebration, FL, United States.

[3] Medical Wellness Advent Health Celebration, FL, United States.

[4] University of South Florida, Tampa, FL, United States.

performing tasks of daily living, and also presents a significant safety concern. Hearing loss presents primarily in two different forms — sensorineural hearing loss and conductive hearing loss, and can also present as a mix of both. There are many causes of hearing loss including, but not limited to, noise exposure, trauma, ototoxic medications, viral infections, vitamin deficiencies, genetics, and aging. While normal hearing is defined as hearing 20–25 dB or better in both ears, disabling hearing loss is categorized by a 35 dB or greater hearing loss in a person's better ear.[1] Of people greater than 60 years old, over 25% are affected by disabling hearing loss.[1] With many advances in technology, there are now ways to help people hear better despite hearing loss; however, preventing hearing loss before it occurs remains an important area of research.

While some risk factors for hearing loss are difficult to alter including genetic causes or certain ear-altering conditions such as noise exposure, ototoxic medications, or Meniere's disease, there are some lifestyle, diet, and supplementary modifications that can be made to potentially mitigate hearing loss.

Noise-induced hearing loss is a form of sensorineural hearing loss that is due to chronic noise exposure. Our world is becoming increasingly inundated with noise — music from speakers, noise from surrounding construction, social environments, music from earbuds, talking on the phone — the list continues. Occupational noise exposure also presents a major concern, and it can be seen in occupations including construction, the military, factory work, and many more. Proper ear protection is critical to preventing occupational hearing loss; however, improper usage of ear protection significantly decreases the potential benefits. Early detection is critical in these occupations to decrease further decline in hearing, routine screening in these occupational environments where noise exposure is common can help to identify individuals and provide appropriate treatment quickly.

Noise exposure at or above 85 dB is known to contribute to a permanent threshold shift (PTS) and results in changes to the sensory structures in the organ of Corti.[2] Additionally, according to the World Health Organization, over 1 billion young adults are at risk of hearing loss due to unsafe listening practices.[1] One study revealed that adolescents who used earphones in a noisy environment for more than 80 minutes per day had a 4.7 times increased risk of hearing loss.[2] The same study found that using earphones in a noisy environment and time spent listening with earphones in a noisy environment were significantly associated with hearing loss.[2] In a noisy environment, one usually wants to "block out" the noise with music; however, it may be doing us more harm in the long-run. Instead, there are many safe alternatives to counteracting loud or annoying sounds such as noise cancelling headphones, white noise devices, earmuffs, and earplugs. While one might not consider that exercising can contribute to noise-induced hearing loss, a wind tunnel experiment that looked at wind tunnel noise experienced by cyclists revealed that wind turbulence, which can get to over 100 dB, can contribute to noise-induced hearing loss.[3]

Smoking seems to be a major risk factor for just about everything, including hearing loss. There appears to be a dose-dependent relationship between smoking and noise-induced hearing loss.[4] Smoking also has a well-established association with otitis media in infants. Chronic otitis media in childhood is also a known cause of hearing loss.[1] Intrauterine infections, meningitis and other infections in childhood are also known causes of hearing loss.[1] These include the "TORCH" infections and without treatment the prevalence can be as high as 28%.[5] Early identification and treatment will limit the impact on the individual. Additionally, following appropriate immunization schedules is important as many of these infections are largely preventable with vaccines.[1] The prevalence of vaccine preventable infections remains high worldwide. Congenital rubella is one of the major preventable causes of hearing loss globally. Proper vaccination before child-bearing age in women could substantially if not almost entirely eliminate cases.[5]

Medications Proposed for Hearing Loss

Noise exposure is known to reduce free magnesium in the serum and perilymph due to a stress-related increase in free fatty acids which binds to free magnesium.[6] One study looked at young healthy individuals who underwent basic military training and were exposed to high levels of impulse noise with ear plugs.[6] Subjects in the treatment arm were given magnesium supplementation, while others received a placebo.[6] It was found that magnesium supplementation prophylactically reduced noise-induced permanent threshold shifts.[6] Magnesium is also known to be a glutamate antagonist and there is evidence that glutamate receptor antagonism affects auditory sensitivity and also possibly tinnitus.[7] Ear protection is important in high noise exposure environments; however, they need to be worn properly in order to exhibit a protective effect. Magnesium supplementation potentially presents a useful way of protecting hearing even when using ear protection.

There is a specific class of drugs that have been shown to attenuate the effect of loud noise on hearing loss referred to as lazaroids.[8] These drugs function through scavenging of free radicals and inhibition of lipid peroxidation.[8] Even in ischemic conditions, this drug class has been shown to stabilize membranes and maintain vitamin E levels, another important contributor to audiologic health.[8] Minor venous irritation has been the only significant side effect known to date.[8] These studies demonstrate possible treatment for noise-induced hearing loss as well as other inner ear pathologies that are related to vascular insult or ischemia.

Further, additional studies on mice showed that polyethylene glycol and allopurinol may preserve cochlear sensitivity after noise exposure causing a threshold shift.[9] The mice in one experimental group were treated with polyethylene glycol, while a separate treatment group was treated with allopurinol and were compared with controls.[9] The results showed statistically significant lower threshold shifts than the controls demonstrating the ability of these two medications to have a protective effect on the cochlea.[9] An additional study also demonstrated the same effect when animals were treated with superoxide dismutase. It is important to note, however, that none of these studies demonstrated cochlear sensitivity returning to baseline after acoustic insult.[9]

Acoustic trauma and exposure to ototoxins principally affect sensory hair cells via the MAP kinase (MAPK) cell death signaling pathway.[10] The MAPK–JNK signal pathway is associated with injury and blocking of this signal pathway prevents apoptosis in areas of aminoglycoside damage.[10] D-JNKI-1 is a cell-permeable peptide that blocks the MAPK–JNK signal pathway and prevents acoustic trauma-induced permanent hearing loss in a dose-dependent manner when delivered locally.[11] D-JNKI-1 completely prevented hair cell death initiated by neomycin exposure to organ of Corti explants, and results from *in vivo* studies showed that direct application of D-JNKI-1 into the scala tympani prevented nearly all hair cell death and permanent hearing loss induced by neomycin ototoxicity.[11] Therefore, D-JNKI-1 is of potential therapeutic value for long-term protection of both the morphological integrity and physiological function of the organ of Corti during times of oxidative stress.

It has been suggested that the initiation phase of cochlear tinnitus is dependent on N-methyl-D-aspartate (NMDA) receptor activity in primary auditory neurons.[12] Esketamine is the *s*-enantiomer of ketamine also known as AM-101. It is a well-known anesthetic and analgesic with selective NMDA receptor antagonism that was developed for treatment of acute inner ear tinnitus.[12] Cochlear NMDA receptors are located at the inner hair cell postsynapse and upregulated after events such as acoustic trauma or hypoxia which cause glutamate excitotoxicity. Glutamate plays a neurotropic role via the activation of NMDA receptors during the process of neosynaptogenesis. It has been proposed that during this critical process of regrowth and synaptic repair of auditory dendrites, the auditory nerve may be particularly susceptible to (aberrant) excitation via NMDA receptors thus generating "phantom noise."[12] AM-101 aims to treat tinnitus in the acute stage before it becomes centralized or memorized at higher structures of the auditory system. It is delivered in a hyaluronic acid gel formulation by injection into the middle ear allowing for highly targeted cochlear therapy with only minimal systemic exposure.[12]

Genetics and Ototoxic Medications

Although primary prevention can be extremely effective, there is also secondary prevention to slow the progression of hearing loss and limit the effects on the individual in children with congenital hearing loss. Secondary prevention is critical to children who would have an effect on their development and school performance if the intervention window passes. Therefore, early detection is essential and can be achieved through routine newborn hearing screening tests.[6] Early detection should not be limited to only the youth either. Hearing loss has been shown to be independently associated with dementia as the severity of hearing impairment has a direct relationship with the likelihood of dementia.[6] Therefore, hearing impairment can be used as a screening for impending cognitive dysfunction in aging adults demonstrating the necessity for early identification in the elderly as well.[6]

Another way to prevent hearing loss is through avoidance of known ototoxic medications. Some known ototoxic medications include aminoglycosides, macrolides, salicylates, NSAIDs, loop diuretics, antimalarials, acetaminophen, and some chemotherapeutic agents like cisplatin.[13] Ototoxic medications are known to cause a bilateral sensorineural hearing loss affecting the higher frequencies of hearing.[13] Ototoxicity results in cellular damage to the inner ear that is irreversible in nature.[13] These medications, while potentially harmful to all patients exposed, can be particularly damaging in patients who already experience some hearing loss. Practitioners should be aware of the ototoxic side effects of these medications before prescribing them, being sure to weigh the alternatives and the potential risks to hearing. Ototoxic effects of aminoglycosides are particularly amplified in people with a certain genetic mutation that has been identified in Caucasian, Chinese, and Japanese individuals, as well as a large Balinese family pedigree.[14] The mutation is an A1555G point mutation in a highly conserved mitochondrial DNA gene that predisposes individuals to sensorineural deafness when exposed to aminoglycosides.[14]

The membrane hypothesis of aging proposes an association between reactive oxygen species, mitochondrial DNA damage, and the aging process. The body continuously creates toxins known as free radicals that are responsible for aging in many parts of the body including the ear in a process known as presbycusis. As we age, the production of these free radicals increases and speeds aging, which includes hearing loss. It has been well documented throughout the literature that increasing the body's antioxidant defenses against oxidative stress is an effective way to slow the progression of age-related damage to the body. Therefore, enhancing the cochlea's antioxidant defense may render the cochlea less susceptible to age-related hearing loss. Oxidative stress markers are being studied as they can help reveal stress in advance of significant damage.[15] The adult hearing loss gene is one such marker and has been associated with increased oxidative stress within cells.[15] The cochlear antioxidant defense has been shown in the literature to be enhanced by endogenous and exogenous treatments.[15]

Endogenous treatment of oxidative stress revolves around increasing the blood flow to the cochlea and excitotoxicity of the neural pathways in the auditory system. Interestingly, an augmented acoustic environment has been shown to prevent age-related sensorineural hearing loss more than a quiet controlled environment.[15] An augmented acoustic environment is a noise level that is clearly audible, but not high enough to cause threshold shift.[15] A non-traumatic noise level increases the antioxidant levels significantly in the cochlea.[15] Additionally, studies done on mice have shown that mice raised in an augmented acoustic environment had a reduced auditory brainstem response, reduced anatomic damage to the cochlea, and enhanced central auditory function.[15] These pre-treatments with lower levels of noise toughen the inner ear and can protect against noise-induced hearing loss.[15] However, the limitation of these studies is that a human's daily sound exposure is somewhere between quiet control conditions and the proper level required for augmented acoustic environment. Therefore, further studies need to be conducted to determine the benefit that a more augmented acoustic environment could provide for age-related sensorineural hearing loss in humans.

Exogenous treatment of oxidative stress has shown that diet also appears to impact our hearing. It has been shown that a caloric dietary restriction of 30% can enhance longevity through reduction in the generation of reactive oxygen metabolites.[16] Certain mitochondrial DNA (mtDNA) deletions are known to contribute to hearing loss and aging in general.[17] Dietary restriction has been shown to reduce the accumulation of mtDNA deletions, providing a protective effect for hearing.[17] There are many different forms of dietary restriction including reducing total caloric intake or intermittent fasting for different amounts of time contributing to an overall calorie deficit. A number of nutritional and vitamin deficiencies have been linked to hearing loss; therefore, replenishing those vitamins and minerals can be beneficial to hearing.[1] There are also a number of studied supplements that have been shown to prevent hearing loss.

Supplements for Hearing Loss

Resveratrol is a polyphenol found naturally in foods like grapes, wine, grape juice, peanuts, cocoa, blueberries, bilberries, and cranberries. Resveratrol has been proven to be an important compound for its effects on aging as well as its prevention of hearing loss. Resveratrol has been shown to protect and prevent hair cell loss and protect the cochlea.[18] Further, Resveratrol prevents the expression of COX-2 (cyclooxygenase 2) and 5 LOX (5 lipoxygenase), an important marker of stress and ischemia, and prevents the creation of ROS, protecting the ear from noise-induced hearing loss.[18]

Vitamin E, also known as tocopherol, is a fat-soluble antioxidant. Often polyunsaturated fatty acids undergo autoxidation. Every free radical that is oxidized will damage three other polyunsaturated fatty acids. Vitamin E stops this process by having the ability to donate hydrogen atoms and terminate the oxidation process.[19] Therefore, vitamin E protects circulating lipoproteins and the stability of cell membranes.[19] While supplements exist, common foods that are high in vitamin E include sunflower seeds, pumpkin, almonds, red bell peppers, peanuts, and avocados.

Many of us are aware of the immune benefits of vitamin C. Vitamin C, also known as ascorbic acid, is a water-soluble antioxidant. Vitamin C is not produced by the human body and therefore is a requirement of dietary intake. Its role in the prevention of free-radical damage includes removal of superoxide, thiol, and hydroxyl radicals.[19] It also has the ability to recycle vitamin E, therefore helping to prevent damage on low-density lipoproteins.[19] Foods high in vitamin C include oranges, bell peppers, tomatoes, broccoli, cauliflower, brussels sprouts and white potatoes.

The B vitamins are very important to many physiological functions in the body. A number of the B vitamins have also been found to be important in preventing hearing loss. Vitamin B1 and vitamin B12 have been shown to attenuate hearing loss.[20] A number of other B vitamins are being studied including vitamin B3, where a causational effect has not yet been proven.[20] Taking a vitamin B complex supplement is recommended as it can prevent hearing loss as well as tinnitus.[20] Some foods that are high in the B vitamins include meat, seafood, poultry, eggs, dairy products, legumes, leafy greens, and seeds.

The cochlea, interestingly, has the highest concentration of zinc in the entire human body.[20] Zinc is an important mineral that may positively affect hearing loss and tinnitus, and zinc supplementation can help maintain the high concentrations that are necessary and found in the cochlea.[20] Zinc in combination with vitamin B3 has been shown to aid with the debilitating symptoms of tinnitus, although the effects on hearing loss are not yet known.[20] Oysters, red meat, nuts, beans, dairy, and poultry are all high in zinc and are healthy additions to protect one's hearing.

Melatonin is primarily well known for its effect on our biological clock and regulation of sleep–wake cycles. However, it also is an important neural antioxidant and free-radical scavenger. Evidence has suggested that melatonin enhances the capacity of many antioxidative enzymes such as superoxide dismutase, glutathione peroxidase, and nitric oxide synthase.[19] Therefore, melatonin is helpful in protecting DNA, membrane lipids and cytosolic proteins from free-radical damage.[19] Foods that are a good source of melatonin include eggs, milk, fish, nuts, goji berries, and tart cherries.

All the cells in our body are formed with cell membranes containing phospholipids that work to regulate what can enter and exit a cell. One of the major components of the phospholipid cell membrane is phosphatidylcholine. One specific type of phosphatidylcholine is called lecithin. In a rat model, lecithin supplementation was found to improve sensitivity to auditory stimuli.[21] Further, lecithin supplementation was protective of mitochondrial energy production in the cochlea and was found to prevent ROS-mediated mtDNA damage.[21] As discussed earlier, reactive oxygen species (ROS) production and damage to mtDNA are known causes of hearing loss; therefore, compounds preventing ROS production and preventing mtDNA damage might be protective of hearing.

Alpha lipoic acid and N-acetyl cysteine are two powerful antioxidants that, in a rat model, have been shown to protect hair cells and prevent presbycusis.[22,23] N-acetyl cysteine is a compound that seeks out and eliminates ROS, an important known contributor to hearing loss.[23] These compounds are also studied for their efficacy in chronic diseases and cognitive decline and they are readily sold as supplements. Coenzyme Q10 (CoQ10) is another powerful antioxidant that has been shown in a small trial to alleviate tinnitus in those with low CoQ10 blood levels prior to starting the supplement.[24] Another study found that CoQ10 may help attenuate hearing loss associated with mitochondrial DNA mutations.[25]

Additionally, there are a number of supplements that have been used for centuries that have anecdotal evidence for preventing or attenuating hearing loss. While there is little scientific evidence on the benefits of these compounds, the tradition of using these different compounds continues to be passed down for generations. These herbal remedies include ginkgo extract, hydergine, mullein, and black cohosh.[20]

Healthy Living for Healthy Hearing

In addition to diet, exercise also improves and prevents hearing loss. The most significant link between exercise and hearing is improved circulation, which allows oxygen and important nutrients to be delivered to the auditory system. Aerobic exercise provides the greatest benefit to the cardiovascular system and the recommendations to spend at least 30 minutes 5 days a week performing cardiovascular exercise, but in this case, more is always better![26] Exercise is associated with reducing obesity, which also has a relationship to hearing. It has been found that women with a higher BMI throughout adulthood lost more brain tissue in the temporal region, where the auditory system is located than women with a lower BMI.[26] Excess weight has been linked to increasing the production of free radicals as well as harmful growth factors and hormones that can erode brain tissue.[26] Additionally, excess fat can be responsible for atherosclerosis that limits oxygen flow to the auditory system. A study found that obesity had a greater effect on aging than smoking. The study concludes that obesity caused aging 9 years beyond those who were lean.[27] Therefore, maintaining a healthy weight can help to prevent hearing loss associated with accelerated aging.

The greatest enemy to hearing is damage caused by aging. But today noise is a close second as it is estimated that millions of people will experience impaired hearing before middle age even begins. Today's longer life span and our increasingly noisy world increases everyone's risk of hearing loss. Like all chronic conditions, hearing loss takes a personal and public toll. Severe hearing loss has been estimated to have a cost of approximately $300,000 per person throughout lifetime, a great financial toll along with the personal toll of the condition.[26] Further, the World Health Organization estimates that unaddressed hearing loss has an annual global cost of US $980 billion.[1] While economic cost of hearing loss is important, it cannot compete with the emotional tax of hearing loss causing isolation, loneliness, and stigma, emotionally devastating effects on an individual. Adults with hearing loss have a higher rate of unemployment compared to their well-hearing counterparts.[1] While many options exist for people who have hearing loss, including various types of hearing aids, bone conduction hearing devices, and even cochlear implants, the technology still does not perfectly replicate the nuances and precision with which the natural human ear is made to absorb and interpret sounds. The best cure for hearing loss remains prevention. While this is difficult in an increasingly noisy world, there are several tools one can incorporate in order to prevent or attenuate hearing loss, be it lifestyle changes, changes in dietary patterns, or the addition of different vitamins and nutrients.

References

1. World Health Organization. (2021) *Deafness and Hearing Loss*. https://www.who.int/news-room/fact-sheets/detail/deafness-and-hearing-loss.
2. Byeon H. (2021) Associations between adolescents' earphone usage in noisy environments, hearing loss, and self-reported hearing problems in a nationally representative sample of South Korean middle and high school students. *Medicine* **100**(3):e24056. doi:10.1097/MD.0000000000024056.
3. Seidman MD, Wertz AG, Smith MM, *et al*. (2017) Evaluation of noise exposure secondary to wind noise in cyclists. *Otolaryngol Head Neck Surg* **157**(5):848–52. doi:10.1177/0194599817715250.
4. Li X, Rong X, Wang Z, Lin A. (2020) Association between smoking and noise-induced hearing loss: A meta-analysis of observational studies. *Int J Environ Res Public Health* **17**(4):1201. doi:10.3390/ijerph17041201.
5. Brown CS, Emmett SD, Robler SK, Tucci DL. (2018) Global hearing loss prevention. *Otolaryngol Clin North Am* **51**(3):575–92. doi:10.1016/j.otc.2018.01.006. Epub 2018 Mar 7. PMID: 29525388.
6. Attias J, Weisa G, Almog S, *et al*. (1994) Oral magnesium intake reduced permanent hearing loss induced by noise exposure. *Am J Otolaryngol* **15**:26–32.
7. Tolonen M. (1992) *Vitamins and Mineral in Health and Nutrition*. New York: E Horwood.
8. Quirk WS, Shivapuja BG, Schwimmer CL, Seidman MD. (1994) Lipid peroxidation inhibitor attenuates noise-induced temporary threshold shifts. *Hear Res* **74**(1–2):217–20. doi:10.1016/0378-5955(94)90189-9. PMID: 8040090.
9. Seidman MD, Quirk WS, Nuttall AL, Schweitzer VG. (1991) The protective effects of allopurinol and superoxide dismutase-polyethylene glycol on ischemic and reperfusion-induced cochlear damage. *Otolaryngol Head Neck Surg* **105**(3):457–63. doi:10.1177/019459989110500318.

10. Lefebvre PP, Malgrange B, Lallemend F, *et al.* (2002) Mechanisms of cell death in the injured auditory system: Otoprotective strategies. *Audiol Neurootol* **7**(3):165–70. doi:10.1159/000058304.
11. Wang J, Van De Water TR, Bonny C, *et al.* (2003) A peptide inhibitor of c-Jun N-terminal kinase protects against both aminoglycoside and acoustic trauma-induced auditory hair cell death and hearing loss. *J Neurosci* **23**(24):8596–607. doi:10.1523/JNEUROSCI.23-24-08596.2003.
12. van de Heyning P, Muehlmeier G, Cox T, *et al.* (2014) Efficacy and safety of AM-101 in the treatment of acute inner ear tinnitus — A double-blind, randomized, placebo-controlled phase II study. *Otol Neurotol* **35**(4):589–97. doi:10.1097/MAO.0000000000000268.
13. Joo Y, Cruickshanks KJ, Klein BEK, *et al.* (2018) Prevalence of ototoxic medication use among older adults in Beaver Dam, Wisconsin. *J Am Assoc Nurse Pract* **30**(1):27–34. doi:10.1097/JXX.0000000000000011.
14. Malik S, Sudoyo H, Sasmono T, *et al.* (2003) Nonsyndromic sensorineural deafness associated with the A1555G mutation in the mitochondrial small subunit ribosomal RNA in a Balinese family. *J Hum Genet* **48**(3):119–24. doi:10.1007/s100380300018.
15. Bielefeld EC, Tanaka C, Chen GD, Henderson D. (2010) Age-related hearing loss: Is it a preventable condition? *Hear Res* **264**(1–2):98–107. doi:10.1016/j.heares.2009.09.001. Epub 2009 Sep 6. PMID: 19735708; PMCID: PMC2868117.
16. Hanjani NA, Vafa M. (2018) Protein restriction, epigenetic diet, intermittent fasting as new approaches for preventing age-associated diseases. *Int J Prev Med* **9**:58.
17. Seidman MD. (2000) Effects of dietary restriction and antioxidants on presbyacusis. *Laryngoscope* **110**(5 Pt 1):727–38. doi:10.1097/00005537-200005000-00003.
18. Seidman M, Babu S, Tang W, *et al.* (2003) Effects of Resveratrol on acoustic trauma. *Otolaryngol Head Neck Surg* **129**(5):463–70. doi:10.1016/s0194-5998(03)01586-9.
19. Wang X, Quinn PJ. (2000) The location and function of vitamin E in membranes (review). *Mol Membr Biol* **17**(3):143–56. doi:10.1080/09687680010000311. PMID: 11128973.
20. Seidman MD, Babu S. (2003) Alternative medications and other treatments for tinnitus: Facts from fiction. *Otolaryngol Clin North Am* **36**(2):359–81. doi:10.1016/s0030-6665(02)00167-6.
21. Seidman MD, Khan MJ, Tang WX, Quirk WS. (2002) Influence of lecithin on mitochondrial DNA and age-related hearing loss. *Otolaryngol Head Neck Surg* **127**:138–44.

22. Huang S, Xu A, Sun X, *et al.* (2020) Otoprotective effects of α-lipoic acid on A/J mice with age-related hearing loss. *Otolo Neurotol* **41**(6):e648–54. doi:10.1097/MAO.0000000000002643.
23. Marie A, Meunier J, Brun E, *et al.* (2018) N-acetylcysteine treatment reduces age-related hearing loss and memory impairment in the senescence-accelerated prone 8 (SAMP8) mouse model. *Aging Dis* **9**(4):664–73. doi:10.14336/AD.2017.0930.
24. Khan M, Gross J, Haupt H, *et al.* (2007) A pilot clinical trial of the effects of coenzyme Q10 on chronic tinnitus aurium. *Otolaryngol Head Neck Surg,* **136**(1):72–7. doi:10.1016/j.otohns.2006.07.010.
25. Angeli SI, Liu XZ, Yan D, *et al.* (2005) Coenzyme Q-10 treatment of patients with a 7445A — G mitochondrial DNA mutation stops the progression of hearing loss. *Acta Otolaryngol* **125**(5):510–2. doi:10.1080/00016480510026232.
26. Moneysmith M, Seidman MD. (2014) *Save Your Hearing Now: The Revolutionary Program That Can Prevent and May Even Reverse Hearing Loss.* New York: Grand Central Publishing.
27. Valdes AM, Andrew T, Gardner JP, *et al.* (2005) Obesity, cigarette smoking, and telomere length in women. *Lancet* **366**(9486):662–4. doi:10.1016/S0140-6736(05)66630-5. PMID: 16112303.

4 Genetic Evaluation for Hearing Loss: Implications for Management

A. Eliot Shearer, MD, PhD[1,2]

Abstract

Hearing loss is a symptom of an underlying pathologic change to the auditory system. Determining the cause of hearing loss is critical for appropriate treatment for children and adults affected by this condition. Because the majority of hearing loss in children is due to a genetic cause, genetic evaluation has become a cornerstone for clinical evaluation and diagnosis. However, because there are hundreds of known hearing loss-associated genes, genetic testing for hearing loss is complex. Testing of all known hearing loss genes at once is required for effective and accurate genetic diagnosis — single gene testing is generally ineffective. Determining the etiology for hearing loss provides several important pieces of information to the patient and the clinician, including prognosis, recurrence risk, and evaluation for syndromic forms of hearing loss. Importantly, a genetic diagnosis is required for enrolment in any new and upcoming clinical trials for cellular, molecular, or gene therapies for hearing loss.

Introduction

Hearing loss is the most common sensory deficit in humans occurring in one in 500 births. Hearing loss is a symptom of an underlying pathological change to the auditory system which includes the outer, middle, and inner

Corresponding Author: A. Eliot Shearer, MD, PhD

[1] Department of Otolaryngology–Head and Neck Surgery, Harvard Medical School, Boston, MA, United States.

[2] Department of Otolaryngology and Communication Enhancement, Boston Children's Hospital, Boston, MA, United States.

ear as well as the auditory nerve and brain. Sensorineural hearing loss is due to alterations or damage to the inner ear (cochlea), auditory nerve, or brain. Syndromic hearing loss is characterized by hearing loss co-occurring with other clinical findings (i.e., blindness or vision loss, thyroid abnormalities, or kidney abnormalities). This is in contrast with non-syndromic hearing loss for which hearing loss is the only clinical finding. There are several forms of syndromic hearing loss that present as non-syndromic hearing loss because the syndromic clinical finding has not yet manifested at the time of diagnosis, called non-syndromic mimics (or apparent non-syndromic hearing loss). A classic example is Usher syndrome, the most common cause of genetic deaf-blindness. The vision loss associated with retinitis pigmentosa does not present until later childhood or the teen years and for this reason in young children, Usher syndrome 'mimics' non-syndromic hearing loss. Determining the cause of hearing loss, or etiological diagnosis, has important implications for clinical management of hearing loss.

Globally, about half of childhood hearing loss is genetic but in developed countries like the United States, approximately 65% of childhood hearing loss is due to a genetic cause (Figure 4.1).[1] The genetic contribution to adult hearing loss is lower, between 20 and 40%, although data are more limited. Non-genetic causes of hearing loss include noise exposure, infectious etiologies, ototoxic medications, trauma, and structural abnormalities of the inner ear. Hearing loss is characterized by extreme genetic heterogeneity, as there are hundreds of known hearing loss-associated genes.

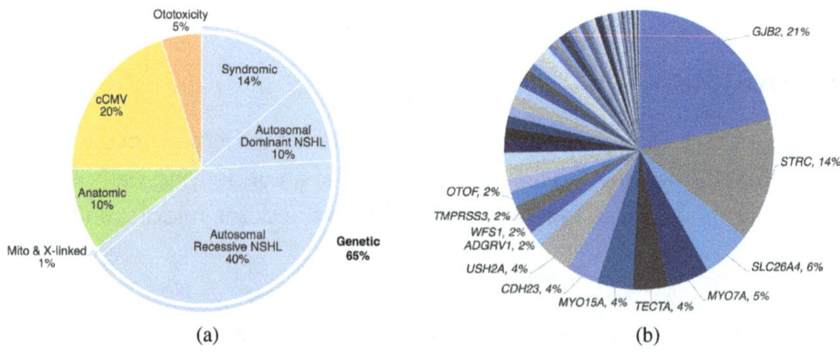

Fig. 4.1 **(a)** Causes of congenital hearing loss, adapted from Morton and Nance[9] and Lieu *et al.*[10] NSHL, non-syndromic hearing loss; cCMV, congenital cytomegalovirus. **(b)** Genetic contribution to hearing loss 2,440 individuals with hearing loss, adapted from Shearer *et al.*[3]

The genetic heterogeneity of hearing loss has historically made genetic testing for this condition difficult. However, determining the genetic cause of hearing loss provides critical information to individuals with hearing loss as well as their healthcare providers. An etiological diagnosis for hearing loss provides information on prognosis (progression of hearing loss over time), recurrence risk, and evaluation for syndromic causes of hearing loss. For these reasons, an etiological diagnosis provides a sense of empowerment for those with hearing loss as it helps to determine the best treatment option. Finally, a genetic diagnosis is required for any available or upcoming clinical trial or clinical use of cellular, molecular, or genetic therapies for hearing loss. This chapter focuses on the most common methods for genetic testing for hearing loss and highlights some key genetic causes of hearing loss.

Methods for Genetic Evaluation

Hearing loss is characterized by extraordinary genetic heterogeneity: more than 120 non-syndromic hearing loss genes with more than 7,000 pathogenic (causative) genetic variations to date. There are more than 400 genes implicated in syndromic hearing loss. An up-to-date list of hearing loss genes and pathogenic hearing loss mutations is maintained online (https://hereditaryhearingloss.org and https://deafnessvariationdatabase.org, respectively).

The most common cause of genetic hearing loss is pathogenic variations in the gene *GJB2* (connexin 26). In some populations, *GJB2* causes up to 50% of genetic hearing loss, but there is significant variation based on genetic ancestry, with White and Asian populations most likely to have *GJB2* as the cause of hearing loss. In mixed ethnic populations, the contribution of *GJB2* is about 20% (Figure 4.1).[2] The second most common cause of genetic hearing loss is pathogenic variants in the gene *STRC*, about 14% of genetic diagnoses. This gene typically causes a mild to moderate form of sensorineural hearing loss. Beyond *GJB2* and *STRC*, no other gene makes up a preponderance of genetic hearing loss. One study showed that in a population of more than 2,000 patients with hearing loss, there were more than 50 different genes involved.[3] This means that testing for a single hearing loss gene is unlikely to be diagnostic.

Genetic testing for hearing loss was revolutionized by the advent of new genetic sequencing technologies that emerged between 2005 and 2010 called next-generation sequencing or massively parallel sequencing. These technologies allow genetic sequencing at an exponentially larger scale than previously available. This allowed, for the first time, in 2010, for comprehensive evaluation of all known hearing loss genes simultaneously.[4] This technology quickly became the standard of care due to greatly increased diagnostic rates compared with single gene testing.[5]

Today, there are several different companies offering 'gene panels' for genetic evaluation of hearing loss. These panels vary with the technology used for genomic sequencing and the exact number of genes included, ranging from dozens to hundreds, but share the goal of evaluating for many hearing loss genes simultaneously. It is important to ensure that a gene panel used for genetic testing for hearing loss is comprehensive, i.e., includes all known hearing loss genes including syndromic forms of hearing loss and includes evaluation for copy number variation, as this is a common cause of *STRC* hearing loss (see below).

Results from hearing loss genetic testing panels typically take 1–3 months and come in the form of a diagnostic report which should be evaluated by a clinician. A medical geneticist or a genetic counsellor will most commonly interpret and return genetic testing results and provide counselling and interpretation of findings. Genetic testing for hearing loss in children is now typically, but not always, covered by private insurance. Prior authorization with an insurance company is recommended.

Important Causes of Genetic Non-Syndromic Hearing Loss

The three genes below were selected for their importance to the field and clinical implications, a basic understanding of these genes will help the practitioner understand the complexity of genetic hearing loss. Given that there are 124 known non-syndromic hearing loss genes and more than 400 reported syndromic forms of genetic hearing loss, these genes below represent only a small proportion of the genetic contribution to hearing loss.

The most common genetic cause of hearing loss overall is *GJB2*, or connexin 26. The protein encoded by this gene forms a crucial ion pore between cells in the organ of Corti. There are hundreds of known pathogenic (causative) variants identified in *GJB2*. *GJB2*-related hearing loss is characteristically bilateral, congenital, and severe to profound. However, hearing loss caused by pathogenic variants in *GJB2* can in fact be quite variable with severity ranging from mild-to-severe to profound and unilateral or bilateral and progressive or stable cases reported.[6] *GJB2* hearing loss may be inherited in autosomal dominant or recessive forms, and is associated with both non-syndromic and syndromic hearing loss. Individuals with *GJB2* hearing loss may be treated with hearing aids or cochlear implants. Several studies have shown that cochlear implants are especially effective for those with hearing loss due to *GJB2* compared to other forms of genetic hearing loss.[7]

Pathogenic variants in the gene *STRC* are the second most common cause of non-syndromic hearing loss overall.[2] *STRC* causes autosomal recessive non-syndromic hearing loss as well as Deafness Infertility Syndrome. *STRC* hearing loss contrasts with *GJB2* hearing loss in that it is mild to moderate and flat in configuration and relatively stable over time. There are some recent data showing very slow progression of *STRC* hearing loss over years. Stereocilin, the protein encoded by *STRC*, functions to tether the outer hair cells of the organ of Corti to the overlying tectorial membrane. The resultant disconnection between these structures causes a mild-to-moderate hearing loss. The importance of *STRC* to genetic hearing loss was not recognized until relatively recently due to the difficulty with genetic sequencing of the *STRC* gene region. This region of the human genome is composed of a tandem genomic duplication — the *STRC* gene and surrounding genomic area is duplicated and the duplicated version of the gene has been inactivated through a stop mutation. The *STRC* duplication makes this area of the genome especially vulnerable to genomic rearrangements that lead to large gene deletions and duplications and makes genetic sequencing very challenging. *STRC* gene deletions may also involve the nearby gene *CATSPER2*. The *CATSPER2* gene is integral to sperm motility and so a homozygous genomic deletion that involves *STRC* and *CATSPER2* results in Deafness Infertility Syndrome in males. *STRC*-associated hearing loss is typically treated with hearing aids given the mild-to-moderate severity.

The most common genetic cause of auditory neuropathy spectrum disorder are mutations in the gene *OTOF*.[8] This gene is of particular contemporary importance, given that it is the target of early human clinical trials for gene therapy. Auditory neuropathy occurs when there is ineffective transfer of neural signal from the inner hair cell of the organ of Corti via the auditory nerve to the brain. Diagnosis of auditory neuropathy is characterized by functional outer hair cells (normal otoacoustic emissions, OAE) and abnormal auditory brainstem response (ABR). The *OTOF* gene encodes otoferlin, a protein that is responsible for tethering of vesicles that release glutamate from the inner hair cells of the organ of Corti. This means that the transmission of auditory stimuli from inner hair cells to the auditory nerve is inhibited. *OTOF*, like other auditory neuropathy spectrum disorders, is associated with variable presentation of hearing loss and includes bilateral, asymmetric, unilateral, and fluctuating hearing loss that may be mild to severe. These patients typically do well with cochlear implants. *OTOF* is the target of the first clinical trials for gene therapy for hearing loss. This is primarily because there is a specific known target for gene therapy and the structures necessary for hearing (inner hair cells, neurons) are present.

Conclusion

New methods for genetic evaluation of hearing loss have revolutionized care for those with hearing loss. By understanding the underlying cause of hearing loss, the affected patient and the clinician are provided with valuable information regarding prognosis and treatment options.

References

1. Sheffield AM, Smith RJH. (2019) The epidemiology of deafness. *Cold Spring Harb Perspect Med* **9**(9):a033258. doi:10.1101/cshperspect.a033258.
2. Sloan-Heggen CM, Bierer AO, Shearer AE, *et al.* (2016) Comprehensive genetic testing in the clinical evaluation of 1119 patients with hearing loss. *Hum Genet* **135**(4):441–50. doi:10.1007/s00439-016-1648-8.
3. Shearer AE, Shen J, Amr S, *et al.* (2019) A proposal for comprehensive newborn hearing screening to improve identification of deaf and hard-of-hearing children. *Genet Med* **21**(11):2614–30. doi:10.1038/s41436-019-0563-5.

4. Shearer AE, DeLuca AP, Hildebrand MS, *et al.* (2010) Comprehensive genetic testing for hereditary hearing loss using massively parallel sequencing. *Proc Natl Acad Sci* **107**(49):21104–9. doi:10.1073/pnas.1012989107.
5. Shearer AE, Smith RJH. (2015) Massively parallel sequencing for genetic diagnosis of hearing loss: The new standard of care. *Otolaryngol Head Neck Surg* **153**(2):175–82. doi:10.1177/0194599815591156.
6. Snoeckx RL, Huygen PLM, Feldmann D, *et al.* (2005) GJB2 mutations and degree of hearing loss: A multicenter study. *Am J Hum Genet* **77**(6):945–57. doi:10.1086/497996.
7. Shearer AE, Hansen MR. (2019) Auditory synaptopathy, auditory neuropathy, and cochlear implantation. *Laryngoscope Investig Otolaryngol* **4**(4):429–40. doi:10.1002/lio2.288.
8. Rodríguez-Ballesteros M, del Castillo FJ, Martín Y, *et al.* (2003) Auditory neuropathy in patients carrying mutations in the otoferlin gene (OTOF). *Hum Mutat* **22**(6):451–6. doi:10.1002/humu.10274.
9. Morton CC, Nance WE. (2006) Newborn hearing screening — A silent revolution. *New Engl J Med* **354**(20):2151–64. doi:10.1056/nejmra050700.
10. Lieu JEC, Kenna M, Anne S, Davidson L. (2020) Hearing loss in children. *JAMA* **324**(21):2195–205. doi:10.1001/jama.2020.17647.

5 Management of Conductive and/or Mixed Hearing Loss

Maria-Pia Tuset, MD, MSc[1];
Adrien A. Eshraghi, MD MSc, FACS[2]; Mary Daval, MD[1];
Denis Ayache, MD[1,3]

Abstract

Hearing loss can be classified as sensorineural, conductive, or mixed. Sensorineural hearing loss (SNHL) is associated with a dysfunction of the inner ear, auditory nerve, or central hearing pathway. Conductive hearing loss (CHL) is usually due to outer or middle ear involvement hampering the conduction of sound energy from its source to the inner ear. Mixed hearing loss (MHL) is a combination of CHL and SNHL. Proper characterization of the type of hearing loss is the first step to better identify its underlying cause. A lot of causes, congenital or acquired, can be responsible of conductive or MHL. Depending on the cause and the degree of hearing loss, CHL or MHL can be addressed by medical therapy, surgical procedure or conventional or implanted hearing aids.

Introduction

Conductive hearing loss (CHL) happens when the transmission of sound waves from their origin to the inner ear sensory cells is hampered. Most commonly, the issue is located in the outer or middle ear (Figure 5.1). However, in some cases, inner ear disease can present itself as CHL or mixed hearing loss (MHL), combining mechanical and sensorineural mechanisms.

Corresponding Author: Ayache Denis MD

[1] Department of Otolaryngology–Head and Neck Surgery, Adolphe de Rothschild Foundation Hospital, Paris, France

[2] University of Miami Miller School of Medicine, Miami, FL, United States

[3] College of Medicine of Paris Hospital

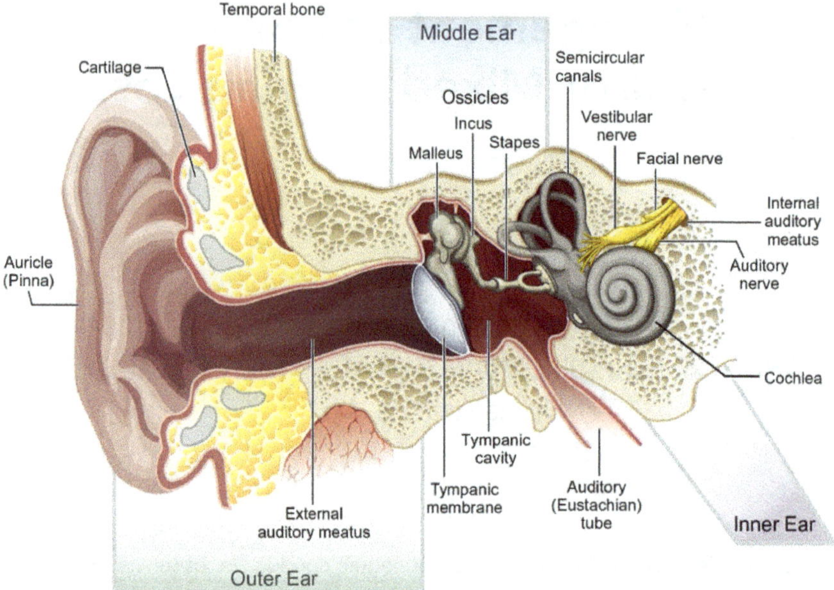

Figure 5.1 Coronal plane view of the anatomical structures of the outer, middle, and inner ear.

Diagnosis and Management

Hearing loss is assessed through a complete physical examination focusing on otoscopy, tuning fork tests, and pure-tone audiometry measuring air- and bone-conduction hearing thresholds along with word or speech discrimination.

Tuning fork tests will help determine the location and nature of any hearing loss detected. In cases of CHL, the defective or most defective ear hears the sound louder (Weber test) and bone conduction (BC) is better heard than air conduction (AC) (Rinne test).

Otoscopy evaluates external auditory canal (EAC) and tympanic membrane (TM). Pneumatic otoscopy can be helpful in checking TM and malleus mobility.

Pure-tone audiometry evaluates level and type of patient's hearing loss. In the case of CHL, AC thresholds are altered while BC thresholds are normal. In MHL both AC and BC are altered, with AC more than BC. The difference between air and bone-conduction hearing thresholds is called air–bone gap (ABG) (Figure 5.2).

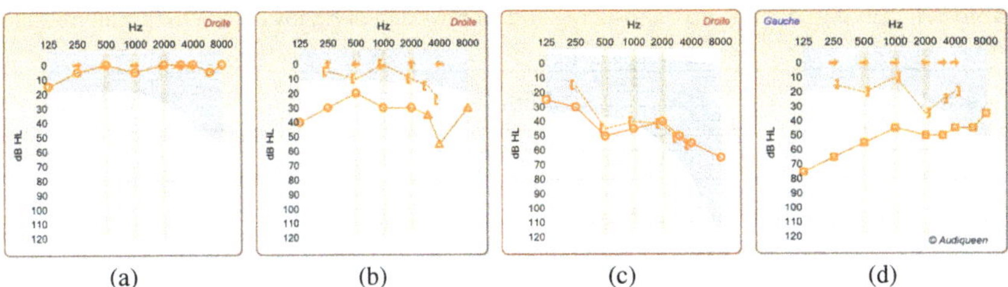

Figure 5.2 **(a)** Audiograms presenting normal hearing, **(b)** conductive hearing loss, **(c)** sensorineural hearing loss, and **(d)** mixed hearing loss. Credit: Rémy Mony, graphic designer.

Once CHL has been diagnosed, the underlying cause needs to be determined. Etiological diagnosis relies on physical examination and in some cases further testing (full audiometry, electrophysiological tests, imaging) is necessary. All etiologies are summarized in Table 5.1, and are explained in more detail in the following subchapters.

The physician first explores the patient's medical history, including any cases of deafness in the family, previous otologic, nasopharyngeal disease and trauma. Accompanying symptoms such as ear pain (otalgia), external ear discharge (otorrhea), external ear bleeding (otorrhagia), tinnitus, or vertigo are noted.

Clinical examination by otoscopy looks for outer ear canal obstruction and allows careful examination of the eardrum (normal, retraction, perforation, bleeding, effusion). Otoscopic examination is performed using a standard otoscope, an otoendoscope, or a binocular microscope. New technologies allowing for otoscopic examination using smartphones and specialized apps are emerging allowing remote consultations.

Pure-tone audiometry, other than differentiating CHL from MHL, is also used to determine the degree of hearing loss. Speech-audiometry testing also explores the severity of the disease but is mostly useful in assessing speech understanding. These are called subjective tests as they solely rely on patients' answers. In children, depending on the age, behavioral tests can be used. These subjective audiometric tests can be completed with objective tests such as tympanometry (Figure 5.3), stapedial reflex evaluation, or electrophysiological tests such as otoacoustic emissions or auditory brainstem responses.

Temporal bone imaging is often performed in the context of trauma, malformation, tumors, chronic otitis media (COM), or conductive/mixed

Table 5.1 Etiologies causing conductive and/or mixed hearing loss in the external, middle, and inner ear.

External ear	Middle ear	Inner ear
Ear wax accumulation	Inflammatory and acute causes: • Acute otitis media • Eustachian tube dysfunction	Semi-circular canal dehiscence
Osteomas, exostoses	Chronic otitis media: • Otitis media with effusion • Chronic otitis media without cholesteatoma (tympanic perforation, ossicular chain damage, tympanosclerosis, atelectatic otitis) • Chronic otitis media with cholesteatoma	Labyrinthine gusher
Acute otitis externa	Otosclerosis	Congenital malformations
Tumors	Trauma	Meniere's and hydropic ear disease
	Congenital malformations	
	Tumors (paragangliomas, schwannomas)	

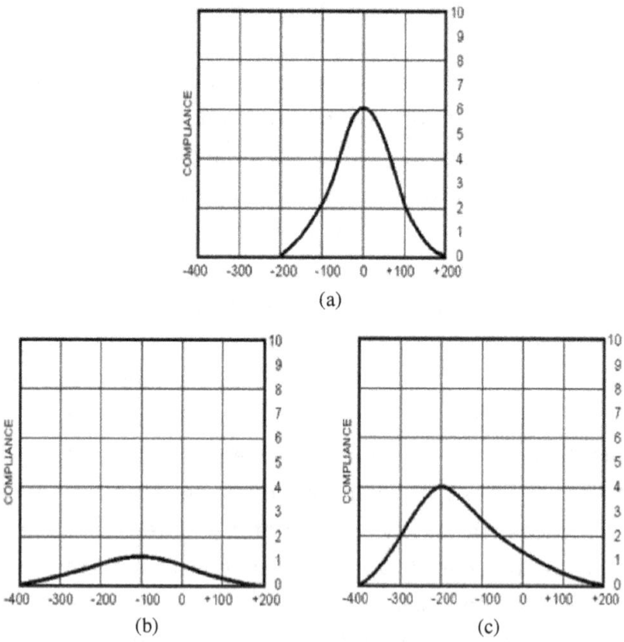

Figure 5.3 **(a)** Tympanograms in a normal ear, **(b)** an ear with eustachian tube dysfunction, and **(c)** an ear with middle ear effusion. Credit: Rémy Mony, graphic designer.

hearing loss (CMHL) with normal TM. In cases of CHL or MHL, thin section non-contrast imaging of the temporal bones with special attention to outer, middle, and inner ear structures, such as high-resolution computed tomography (HRCT) or cone-beam computed tomography (CBCT) is the first-line imaging modality to apply in selected presentations.

Once a diagnosis has been made, disease management will depend on several factors such as the exact cause of hearing loss, its evolution, the risks of the underlying cause, patient's age, and motivation for hearing rehabilitation. Management options are diverse and can be recommended alone or in combination, going from simple surveillance, medical treatments, or surgical treatments. Surgical management is the most common treatment option and entails disease removal or middle ear reconstruction among others. Sound amplification systems using hearing aids (HA) are also valuable treatment options using AC or BC devices. Some of these devices are completely external, while others require surgical placement.

External Ear Pathologies Causing CHL

Ear wax (cerumen) accumulation in the outer ear canal is an extremely frequent cause of ear blockage or CHL, especially when full obstruction of the external auditory canal (EAC) happens. Cerumen impaction is frequent in patients with narrow ear canals, excessive ear canal hygiene, or frequent use of earplugs. Otoscopic examination confirms the diagnosis and careful removal of the impacted cerumen (using cerumenolytic agents, ear irrigation, suction, or special microscopic instruments) allows immediate patient relief and hearing recovery. If any discomfort persists after this a more complete examination including full audiometry is performed.

Osteomas and exostoses of the EAC are benign bony outgrowths narrowing the canal. They can be responsible for CHL in cases of full obstruction of the EAC or when cerumen impaction occurs in the narrowed canal. Most commonly associated with cold water swimming, they are often observed in divers and swimmers. Diagnosis is made after otoscopic examination. When tight strictures are observed and an associated middle ear disease is suspected, computed tomography (CT)-scan examination is recommended. When symptomatic, surgical removal and calibration of the EAC can be performed (canalplasty).

Acute otitis externa is an infection involving the skin of the EAC leading to otalgia, discharge, and CHL from inflammatory stenosis of the EAC. Also termed swimmer's ear, they occur mostly during summer with frequent swimming. Diagnosis is made by otoscopy with careful examination of the tender ear. Otic antibiotic drops and anti-inflammatory medications are usually enough for full recovery, but in painful and very inflamed cases, a small cellulose wick can be placed in the ear canal for a few days.

Tumors of the EAC are quite rare, but when diagnosed they are mostly malignant (squamous cell carcinoma or basal cell carcinomas). They can be revealed by CHL in cases of EAC obstruction, but most frequent symptoms are otalgia (ear pain) or otorrhagia (bleeding from ear). Otoscopic examination and biopsy with histologic analysis are needed for diagnosis. An extensive imaging workup is mandatory to evaluate local and regional tumor extension. Treatment consists in large removal of the lesion with extensive surgery, such as subtotal temporal bone resection with EAC closure, facial nerve sacrifice (rarely), parotidectomy, and reconstruction with myo-cutaneous or free flaps. Supplementary radiotherapy may be needed to complete treatment.

Congenital malformations of the EAC will be explored in another subchapter along with middle ear malformations.

Middle Ear Pathologies Causing CHL

Inflammatory and Acute Causes

Acute otitis media (AOM) are acute infections (<3 weeks) causing inflammation of the middle ear space. Although very common in children they can also occur in adults, after episodes of nasopharyngeal congestion (nasal and back of nose), or sinus inflammation. Symptoms are otalgia, fever, ear discharge, and in some cases CHL. Diagnosis is made after otoscopic examination. Symptomatic treatment of pain and fever are necessary, often in conjunction with oral antibiotic therapy. In cases of mild symptoms, simple surveillance can suffice; in fact when a viral infection is the cause of the disease, spontaneous resolution may occur. Hearing loss will fully recover after successful treatment.

Eustachian tube (ET) dysfunctions occur after rhinitis, nasopharyngitis, or sinusitis. Patients can present hearing loss or aural fullness. Otoscopic examination reveals an inflamed or retracted TM, but the exam may also be normal. Physical examination shows congestion of the nose, throat, or sinus cavities. Valsalva maneuver (forceful exhalation while blocking nose and mouth) may result in transient symptom resolution as it opens the ET. When performed, hearing test may show mild CHL, and tympanometry is altered (Figure 5.3c, type c curve, shifting towards negative pressures). Treatment consists of managing nasal congestion (nose rinsing solutions, decongestant nasal sprays, anti-inflammatory medications, and sometimes antibiotics). Balloon ET dilation or placement of tympanostomy tube may also be an option with appropriate indications.

Chronic Otitis Media

Introduction

Chronic otitis media (COM) refers to all persistent (>6 weeks) inflammations or infections of the middle ear. History of repeated otitis in childhood is often present, but it can occur insidiously.

Although its pathophysiology is still not well understood, many factors are involved: ET dysfunction (its role in middle ear ventilation and drainage if affected leading to depression of the middle ear cavity, TM weakening and mucosal tissue growth with effusion), immune system alterations, and allergies.[1] Patients with cleft palates, Down syndrome, Crouzon syndrome, or metabolic diseases are particularly prone to COM.

Chronic otitis media may clinically present in many ways but always involves chronic inflammation of the middle ear.

Two main types of COM can be distinguished: simple COM, with recurrent drainage and/or hearing loss, or complex and dangerous COMs (mainly represented by cholesteatoma) potentially leading to local or regional severe complications.

Simple COM can occur behind a closed TM and is referred to as otitis media with effusion (OME). It usually resolves without consequences, but can also evolve into adhesive otitis media, tympanic atelectasis (full retraction) or COM with tympanic perforation.

Otitis media with effusion

Otitis media with effusion refers to chronic otitis without perforation of the eardrum, with persistent fluid in the middle ear space. This pathology is common in children between 2 and 4 years old. It is often bilateral and observed during winter and fall. OME is usually associated with repeated nasopharyngeal congestion and otitis media.

Adenoids must certainly play a role in OME (enlarged obstructive adenoids blocking the ET, recurrent nasopharyngeal infection with contiguous ET inflammation). Bilateral hearing loss is the most common symptom, but this changes over time. Aural fullness and autophony (abnormal sound of its own voice) are often reported by adults. Otalgia is rare but when present, an acute infectious episode must be suspected. OME can also be asymptomatic and discovered during routine physical examination.

Depending on the duration of the disease, the TM can present differently: thickened membrane, infiltrated, retracted, inflammatory, with serous fluid effusion, air bubbles, or even bluish in chronic forms. Upon tympanometry the TM can show stiffness with a flat curve. Nasopharyngeal fiberoptic endoscopy is an examination conducted during physical examination. It can be useful in children to assess adenoid volume, search for nasopharyngeal infection signs or gastroesophageal reflux. In adults, it will be mostly used to eliminate the presence of a nasopharyngeal mass, especially when effusion is unilateral. After examination if doubt persists, tympanometry will be performed and show a b type curve reflecting poor mobility of the eardrum thereby suggesting effusion. Audiometry shows CHL, which will vary in severity. This CHL is rarely above 30dB.

Although imaging is usually not recommended in children, it is sometimes needed in adults with chronic or recurring OME evaluation, especially in unilateral cases (evaluate for nose and sinus infection, nasopharyngeal carcinoma, systemic disease, skull base tumors).

In most cases, OME will resolve spontaneously without sequelae, but in a few patients, it will evolve into another form of chronic otitis (adhesive, atelectasis, cholesteatoma).

Medical treatment of OME starts with managing risk factors and inducing factors (treatment of anemia, elimination of tobacco use, nasal hygiene, allergy treatment, and gastroesophageal reflux). Although many treatments have been proposed (antibiotics, steroids, mucolytic agents, decongestants, vaccines, antihistamines), they failed to prove significant efficacy in many cases and the consensus is not clear.[2] Only ET auto inflation devices seem to provide some benefit.

Surgical treatment consists in myringotomy (incision of the eardrum) with ventilation tube (VT) insertion and removal of obstructive adenoids. Adenoidectomy is recommended in cases of recurrent infections, nasal obstruction, or sleep apnea. In cases of prolonged (>3 months) and symptomatic CHL or MHL, (recurrent ear infections, effusion, tympanic retraction such as retraction pockets), VT are inserted into the TM to equalize pressures on each side of the TM and restore proper aeration of the middle ear. Patient guidelines for water penetration will depend on the type of tube used and surgeon's recommendations.

Chronic otitis media without cholesteatoma

Unlike cholesteatoma, which will be discussed in another subchapter, this type of COM can be referred to as 'harmless.' Even if they can bring discomfort to patients through discharge, hearing loss of varying degrees, and swimming restrictions, they do not carry the same risk of complications as cholesteatoma. Nevertheless, these non-cholesteatomatous forms need to be monitored regularly as they can progress to cholesteatoma.[3] They are usually the consequence of active or past inflammations. Otitis media with tympanic perforation is defined by chronic inflammation of the middle ear mucosa with tympanic perforation, leading to recurrent suppurative (mucous or pus) otorrhea, particularly after swimming or after nose and throat infections. Hearing loss of varying degrees is associated especially when otorrhea is present. Otoscopy examination reveals a perforated TM with inflammatory residues, and an inflamed, humid, and thickened middle ear mucosa. Treatment is usually purely medical (ear hygiene, non-ototoxic ear drops) and aims to dry the middle ear cavity. After resolution post-discharge, surgical treatment can be proposed to repair the defect of the TM (tympanoplasty).

Sequelae of simple COM: tympanic membrane perforation, ossicular chain discontinuity

Simple COM is a non-evolving type of otitis. The main symptom is hearing loss [severity varying on the ossicular chain and TM damages, or in cases of association with sensorineural hearing loss (SNHL)], and otorrhea.

The most common form is **tympanic membrane perforation**, diagnosed after otoscopy alone and showing a hole in the TM (Figure 5.4a). Audiometry is recommended to rule out a more severe form (ossicular chain damage, SNHL), which will reveal CHL of 30 dB or less.

Management depends on clinical presentation and the patient's wishes and includes surveillance, hearing aid fitting, or surgery.[4] When surveillance is recommended, the patient will have to avoid water penetrating the ear and promptly treat any nasal and throat infection as they may trigger otorrhea. When handicapping hearing loss is present or when the patient does not wish to have surgery, fitting the patient with HA can be proposed. Sound amplification devices using AC can be used but carries a risk of destabilizing the ear by obstructing the canal, potentially leading to maceration and otorrhea, which will impede proper use of the device temporarily or definitively. BC devices are also an option and can be surgically implanted (BAHA, bonebridge or Osia) or not (using headbands, or adhesives). The gold standard treatment option is tympanoplasty, also called myringoplasty when only the eardrum is concerned by the reconstruction. Different surgical techniques exist to reconstruct damaged TMs depending on the size and location of the perforation, the quality of the remaining membrane, the status of the ossicular chain, and the surgeon's

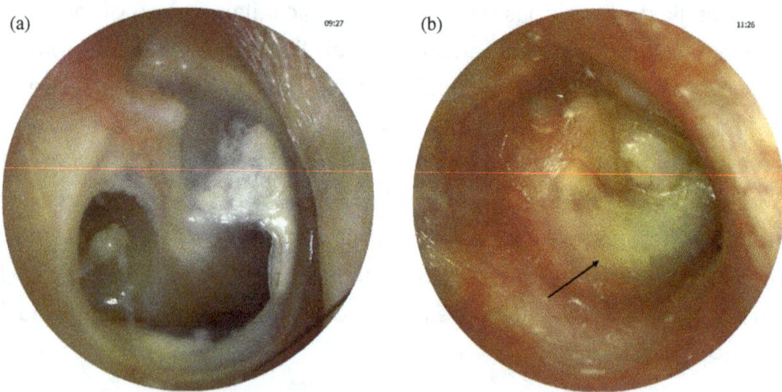

Figure 5.4 Images of right ear tympanic membranes. **(a)** Posterior tympanic membrane perforation. The middle ear cavity is visible through the perforation. Tympanosclerosis is present in the remnant tympanic membrane (white calcifications on the right hand side of the image). **(b)** Reconstructed tympanic membrane with cartilage graft visible posteriorly (black arrow). The graft was placed under the tympanic membrane remnants.

experience. The procedure may be performed under local or general anesthesia in an outpatient surgery facility.

As for all ear surgery, a microscope, exoscope, or endoscope is used for image magnification. TM reconstruction is performed through the EAC (transcanal approach) or through an incision located anteriorly (endaural approach) or posteriorly (retroauricular approach) to the ear canal.

The grafting tissue is harvested from the patient themselves (autograft), from the temporalis fascia, perichondrium, periosteum, cartilage, or adipose tissue. The surgeon elevates a tympanomeatal flap by lifting the skin of the EAC and then the TM. The graft is most often placed under the TM remnants (Figure 5.4b). Techniques using fat tissue or cartilage discs can be positioned through the perforation without elevating a flap. Success rates of myringoplasties range from 75 to 90% depending on age, size, and location of the perforation, and status of the middle ear cavity.[5] Surgical risk is minimal for myringoplasties, but the patient is informed on the surgical risks of any otologic surgery, including: hearing loss, tinnitus, vertigo, taste alterations, and facial nerve palsy.

One of the other sequelae of COM is **ossicular chain discontinuity** (malleus, incus, and stapes) . The ossicular chain transmits sound vibrations to the inner ear fluids. One or more of the ossicles may be eroded, fixed, or both. Erosion of the ossicular chain affects primarily and most frequently the long process of the incus (LPI), but other bones can also be partially or completely eroded. The most common symptom described by patients is hearing loss, often with accompanying tinnitus. Otoscopy examination is performed but is usually not precise enough in identifying the involved ossicle(s). The audiogram shows CHL or MHL with a larger ABG than in TM perforation alone. Temporal bone CT-scan can be helpful in identifying the status of the ossicular chain and location of an eroded ossicle.

Depending on the severity of the hearing loss and its impact on the patient, different approaches are possible. When no hearing impairment exists, simple surveillance is a safe option. When hearing loss is significant, impacting the patient's quality of life, hearing aid fitting, or surgery are proposed. Conventional AC HA as well as non-implantable BC HA or implantable hearing aid devices (BAHA, middle ear implant) can be offered.

Ossiculoplasty, or ossicular chain reconstruction, reestablishes the sound conduction mechanism from the TM to the inner ear fluids. It can be associated with other procedures (myringoplasty, mastoidectomy, cholesteatoma removal) when other structures of the middle ear are also damaged or involved. The surgical approach is similar to that described previously, under general or local anesthesia.

Ossicular chain reconstruction (Figure 5.5) can be performed by harvesting tissue from the patient themselves through surgical incision (Figure 5.5a, ossicular remnant, bony fragment, or a piece of cartilage), by using synthetic prosthesis (Figure 5.5b, c, titanium, hydroxyapatite and Teflon mainly) or by using surgical cement. Three main procedures can be described: partial ossiculoplasty when the stapes is intact and mobile, total ossiculoplasty (Figure 5.5d, e) when the stapes suprastructure is missing with a safe and mobile footplate, and stapes surgery for stapes fixation (stapedectomy or stapedotomy).[6] These techniques are able to resolve pure CHL cases, especially when the middle ear cavity is properly aerated. In cases of MHL, ossicular chain reconstruction corrects the conductive part of hearing (represented by ABG values) but hearing aid fitting is further needed postoperatively to address the remaining sensorineural component.

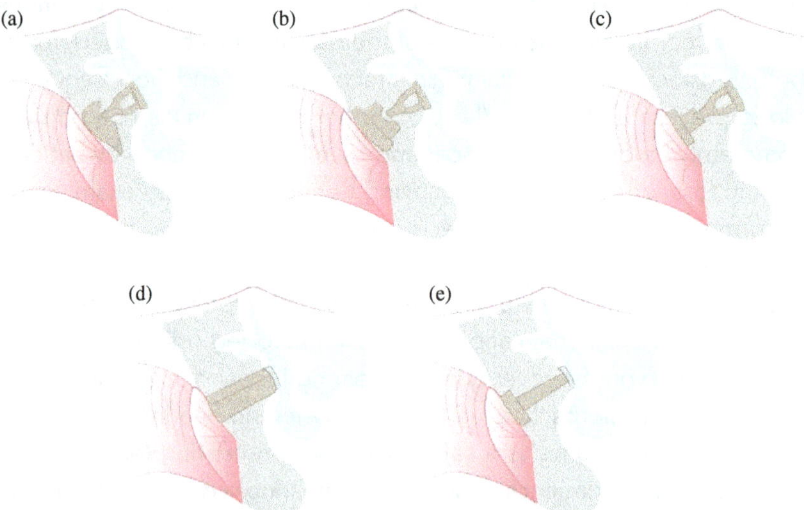

Figure 5.5 Graphical representation of five different types of ossicular chain reconstruction. Partial ossiculoplasties are represented in panel **(a)** (remnant incus), panel **(b)** (cartilage graft), and panel **(c)** (synthetic partial prosthesis). Total ossiculoplasties are presented in panel **(d)** (cartilage) and panel **(e)** (synthetic total prosthesis). Credit: Rémy Mony, graphic designer.

The other forms or sequelae of COM are **tympanosclerosis** (calcified residues frequently found on the TM, causing no harm or extending to the ossicular chain and creating blockage and thereby hearing loss), **fibro-adhesive otitis** (thickened mucosal layer and poor middle ear ventilation, surgery is not often recommended), and **chronic atelectatic otitis**.

Atelectatic otitis needs to be identified and monitored as it is often the starting point to cholesteatoma. This process is secondary to chronic inflammation and weakening of the TM, which, through poor middle ear ventilation, becomes thin, creating a retraction pocket or a complete atelectatic ear.

Otoscopic examination reveals a thin and pellucid eardrum retracted within the middle ear globally or in some areas, creating retraction pockets. Effusion can also be associated. When the condition evolves, surgical treatment is necessary to avoid development of cholesteatoma. Important signs of poor evolution must be known by the physician: retraction pocket not fully controlled (visible) upon otoscopy, presence of skin debris in the retraction pocket, and otorrhea (often because of retraction pocket perforation). These signs must lead to a temporal bone CT-scan to preoperatively check for cholesteatoma and extension. In evolving forms without cholesteatoma, VTs can be placed to limit the progress of the retraction and increase middle ear ventilation, or tympanoplasty for tympanic reinforcement with cartilage graft can be proposed, or both.

COM with cholesteatoma

This type of COM is a serious condition as it has strong potential for erosion and infection and can cause severe complications. Cholesteatomas are benign collections of keratinized squamous epithelium within the middle ear ('wrong skin in the wrong place'). Mostly acquired after recurrent otitis with migration of squamous epithelium from a retraction pocket or tympanic perforation which grows uncontrollably, congenital forms also exist (from an embryonic epithelial tissue remnant within the temporal bone).[7]

The classic presentation is suppurative and foul odor otorrhea and/or variable hearing loss. Unfortunately, sometimes, the disease can also be diagnosed when a complication happens (vertigo, facial nerve paralysis, labyrinthitis, meningitis). Diagnosis can also be made upon routine ear examination in asymptomatic forms.

Physical examination reveals (Figure 5.6): cholesteatoma of the attic (superior cavity of the ME), uncontrollable retraction pocket filled with epidermic debris, sentinel aural polyp hiding attic cholesteatoma, tympanic perforation with visualization of squamous epithelium often infected, a white 'pearly' mass behind an intact eardrum (particularly in congenital cholesteatomas). Associated symptoms should be addressed during initial examination.

Audiometry during initial screening can be normal or show conductive or MHL, or even SNHL when a complication involves the inner ear.

Workup for cholesteatoma includes temporal bone CT-scan. The preoperative CT-scan allows the clinician to evaluate extension of the disease and search for clinically hidden complications and details the anatomy of the tympanic and mastoid cavities. In cases presenting with atypical symptoms, it also helps in confirming the diagnosis.[7,8] Before primary surgery a magnetic resonance imaging (MRI) is rarely useful.

Complications of cholesteatoma come from their strong bony erosion potential and from infection: infectious episodes with otorrhea and otalgia, hearing loss (conductive, mixed, or sensorineural), facial nerve paralysis, vertigo and dizziness (from labyrinthine fistula particularly of the semicircular canal), meningitis, abscess (cerebral or cerebellar), and thrombosis (inflamed blood vessels and/or blood clots) of the sigmoid sinus. Because of its aggressiveness, its management is always based on surgery. The aim

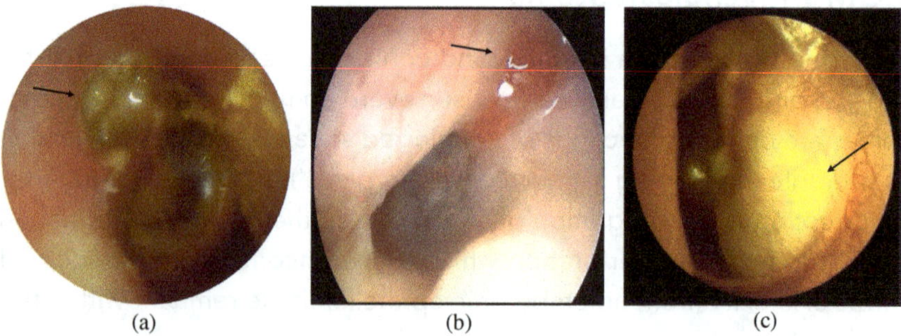

Figure 5.6 Images of tympanic membranes. **(a)** Cholesteatoma of the attic (black arrow) in a right ear. Superior perforation filled with infected epidermic debris. **(b)** Sentinel aural polyp hiding attical cholesteatoma in a left ear (black arrow). **(c)** White 'pearly' mass behind an intact tympanic membrane in a left ear (black arrow).

is complete removal of the mass and recovery of a disease-free, stable, and dry ear, thus avoiding any residual or recurrent cholesteatoma. The second goal of surgery is preserving or improving the patient's hearing. The procedure is performed under general anesthesia in outpatient care. Facial nerve monitoring is conducted throughout surgery. Cholesteatomas limited to the middle ear can be approached using transcanal access with a microscope or an endoscopic ear surgery approach. Extended cholesteatomas are usually approached retroauricularly since it allows access to both the mastoid and middle ear. Several techniques exist (intact canal tympanoplasty with or without mastoid obliteration, canal wall down tympanoplasty with or without canal wall reconstruction and mastoid obliteration).[9–11]

The technique will be chosen depending on which one offers the best chances of full removal in safe conditions. Once cholesteatoma has been removed, the tympanoplasty with primary ossiculoplasty is performed if the surgical conditions are favorable. An operated cholesteatoma must be monitored for many years since the rate of recurrent disease can reach 10%.[12]

Otoscopic examination is essential to assess recurrence but is not enough. In fact, residual disease can often be found behind a cartilage graft or in the mastoid cavity. To avoid any undiagnosed residual disease, a second look surgery can be proposed 1 year after the initial intervention. This will allow full mastoid and middle ear cavity assessment with ossicular chain reconstruction if not performed primarily. Currently, many surgical teams prefer MRI surveillance using specific sequences (diffusion-weighed), recently proven to allow safe and efficient residual and recurrent disease.[13,14]

Otosclerosis

Otosclerosis is a disease characterized by abnormal bone remodeling of the otic capsule (osteodystrophy). Dysplastic bone foci can develop in different locations of the middle and inner ear. Stapes footplate fixation is the most common anomaly observed in patients with otosclerosis, explaining conductive or MHL. Sensorineural disease can be found when the bony foci develop in the inner ear but is rare.[15] Although sporadic cases exist, there is a strong genetic component since family history of otosclerosis exists in 50% of patients. Females are most often concerned (2/1 ratio) and symptoms are usually triggered or aggravated by hormonal factors (pregnancy, contraception). Diagnosis is usually made in patients between 25 and 45 years of age, but may be seen in younger (juvenile otosclerosis) or older patients. Disease is bilateral in close to 75% of cases and disease incidence, represented by hearing loss, ranges from 0.1 to 2%. Nevertheless, temporal bone studies have shown that histological prevalence is much higher, reaching 12% and that patients with silent otosclerotic foci were observed 8–10× more frequently than patients with hearing impairment. It is hypothesized that external factors (viral infections, trauma, hormones) may trigger otosclerosis in genetically prone patients.

There are two main symptoms of otosclerosis: progressive CHL and tinnitus. Vestibular symptoms (dizziness, vertigo, balancing problems) are rare, and require that the physician rules out manières or superior semicircular canal dehiscence. Otoscopy reveals a normal eardrum and tuning fork tests suggests conductive or MHL. Audiometry testing shows CHL with thresholds increasing gradually and an ABG growing larger with stapes fixation. Association with an abnormal BC will result in MHL, most observed as disease progresses. A pure SNHL from otosclerosis is rare and referred to as cochlear otosclerosis. TM compliance is normal, and the stapes reflex is absent as the stapes is immobile.

Temporal bone CT-scan or CBCT shows otosclerotic foci (hypodense foci of the bone surrounding the inner ear), look for a differential diagnosis, and assess for any important anatomical consideration for surgery. As the diagnosis is confirmed by stapes fixation intraoperatively, imaging is not formally recommended by all surgeons before surgery and will depend on the clinical and audiological presentation.[16]

Other causes of CHL and MHL can mimic otosclerosis and should be identified before any surgical procedure is performed, particularly stapes surgery as there is a risk of complications and failure. Congenital or acquired pathologies of the ossicular chain or the middle ear can mimic otosclerosis (labyrinthine malformation, enlarged vestibular aqueduct, enlarged internal auditory canal, superior semicircular canal dehiscence).

Hearing rehabilitation relies on stapes surgery or hearing aid fitting. Medical treatment using sodium fluoride or bisphosphonates can be useful in some patients, especially in cases of aggressive sensorineural disease, to slow disease progression, but efficacy still needs to be demonstrated.

Whenever possible, the preferred treatment by the patient is stapes surgery, to replace the fixed stapes by a prothesis from the incus to the labyrinthine fluid after fenestration (stapedotomy) or removal of the footplate (stapedectomy) and to recover sound transmission to the inner ear fluids (Figure 5.7). Surgery is proposed to patients with CHL or MHL with a minimal ABG of 25–30 dB. In cases of bilateral disease, surgery will be performed on the "worse" hearing ear first. The procedure is performed under general or local anesthesia, in an outpatient setting. A tympanomeatal flap is elevated using the transcanal approach, and the surgeon aims to obtain full exposure of the oval window region. The incus will be separated from the stapes and a calibrated fenestration (stapedotomy) of the footplate will be performed using a perforator, drill, or laser. Total or partial removal of the stapes footplate may sometimes be performed (stapedectomy) followed by using tissue graft for sealing. A stapes prothesis will be placed in the fenestrated footplate and attached to the long process of the incus (LPI). Prosthesis can be made in different materials (fluoroplastic, stainless, titanium) with equivalent results. Placement of the prosthesis using a robotic arm is currently being assessed in clinical research. Results are excellent with a success rate of close to 90% in hearing improvement.[17] A small risk of complications exists (increase of hearing loss severity, may be profound, facial nerve injury, taste disturbance, tinnitus, dizziness) and the patient must be clearly informed.

The alternative option of hearing aid fitting is the other option available to patients declining surgery or in case of surgical contraindication (significant medical conditions not compatible with anesthesia, total hearing loss in the contralateral ear, cochlear otosclerosis, associated malformation of the labyrinth, patient with history of hydrops). HA can also be used to

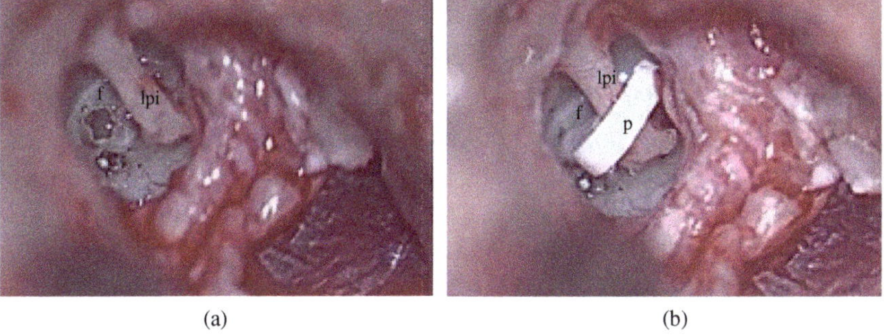

Figure 5.7 Pre-operative images of stapes surgery. The tympanomeatal flap is lifted allowing visualization of the long process of the incus (LPI), and the footplate (f). **(a)** Image of stapedotomy. The stapes has been removed and a hole in the footplate performed. **(b)** Stapedial prosthesis (p) placed on the LPI and lying on the footplate perforation.

complement surgery in patients with MHL and persistent SNHL after successful ABG closure (surgery only addresses the conductive component).

Implantable BC devices or middle ear implants can be discussed in selected cases. In cases of advanced otosclerosis stapedotomy with HA or cochlear implantation can be proposed.[18] This is discussed in more detail in the Cochlear Implant chapter.

Middle Ear Trauma

Tympanic membrane perforations and ossicular chain traumas (fracture and/or dislocation of the ossicles) represent most middle ear trauma cases. They can be secondary to temporal bone fracture or direct trauma from a penetrating foreign body (Q-tip), barotrauma (sudden ambient pressure changes such as from diving or flying resulting in high pressure differentials), or auricular blast (explosion, slapping).

Initial evaluation consists in otoscopy, audiogram, and CT-scan of the temporal bone to evaluate ossicular chain damage.

Traumatic tympanic perforations on a previously normal membrane heal spontaneously in most cases and regular surveillance until healing is recommended. A myringoplasty is indicated when perforation persists 4–6 months after trauma, or when the edges of the TM perforation enter the middle ear cavity risking evolution towards cholesteatoma.

Ossicular chain traumas include dislocations (incudo-stapedial, incudomalleolar, or stapediovestibular) and more rarely fractures (stapes, LPI or malleus).[19] The only surgical emergency is stapediovestibular dislocation, accompanied by vertigo and mixed or SNHL, especially when a tympanic perforation is associated. Hearing rehabilitation is achieved through hearing aid fitting or ossicular chain reconstruction (total or partial depending on ossicular damage). A common but highly underestimated cause of ossicular trauma, particularly of malleus trauma, comes from introduction and brisk withdrawal of a finger in the EAC. When an isolated malleus fracture is present, we prefer reconstruction using surgical cement.

Congenital Malformations of the External and Middle Ear

Congenital malformations of the external ear can be isolated or part of a malformative syndrome (Treacher Collins, Goldenhar, Crouzon syndromes, among others) needing multidisciplinary evaluation. They can concern the auricle (microtia) and/or the EAC (aural atresia or hypoplasia).[20] These types of malformations present functional and aesthetic challenges. Functional deficit is represented by CHL reaching up to 60 dB. Management of the pathology is conducted by highly specialized teams. Hearing rehabilitation can include implantable BC devices or surgery (canalplasty, ossiculoplasty, and/or auricular reconstruction), but surgical correction is often not the preferred treatment as the hearing outcome is no better than those afforded by BC devices, and surgery may be associated with recurrence or complications (meatal stenosis).

Middle ear malformations may involve the ossicles (presenting ankylosis or malformation) or the oval or round window (atretic or hypoplastic). Patients carrying these malformations will have CHL and a normal TM. Ossiculoplasty or hearing aid fitting (conventional or implantable) is the treatment option in these cases.[20]

Tumors of the External and Middle Ear

Tumors are a rare cause of CHL. They can be benign (paragangliomas, schwannomas, adenomas) or malignant in a few cases. Tympanic or tympano-jugular paragangliomas are slow growing, benign vascular tumors arising from paraganglionic cells distributed along the parasympathetic nerves. Some paragangliomas can be associated with other types of lesions (thyroid tumors, pheochromocytoma). In the ear, they can be limited to the middle ear or extend to the jugular foramen and the skull base. Before developing CHL or MHL, the most frequent symptom is pulsatile tinnitus. The diagnosis is suspected after otoscopic examination revealing a reddish and pulsatile middle ear mass (Figure 5.8). Examination is completed by imaging including HRCT of the temporal bones and MRI with vascular sequences. When paragangliomas are limited to the middle ear, surgical removal is conducted. In cases of extension to the jugular foramen or the skull base, surgical resection after preoperative embolization or radiotherapy to stop disease progression is considered.

Facial nerve schwannomas are extremely rare and can develop in the middle ear. Progressive CHL with normal otoscopy and/or progressive and peripheral facial paralysis are observed upon examination. Several factors impact treatment options (patient age, tumor extension, facial paralysis

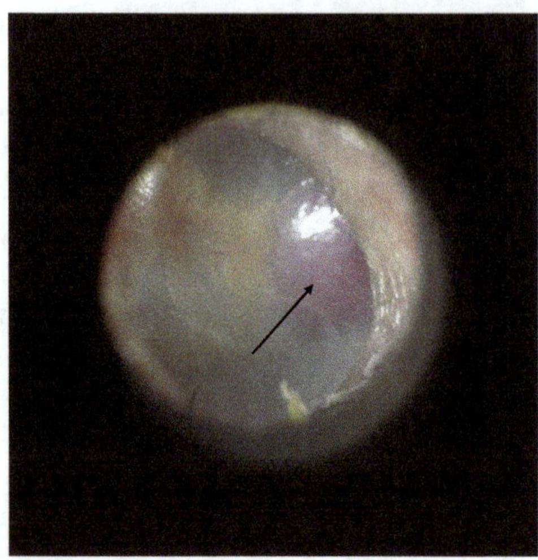

Figure 5.8 Reddish mass behind an intact tympanic membrane (black arrow), revealing a tympano-jugular paraganglioma.

severity), which range from simple surveillance to surgical resection with facial paralysis rehabilitation, or radiotherapy.

Malignant tumors of the ear are rare but carry poor prognosis as they typically present in an advanced stage. Squamous cell carcinoma is the most common type, arising from the auricle or the EAC. Disease symptoms include chronic otorrhea with bleeding, CHL, otalgia, and facial paralysis. Treatment consists of extended resection of the tumor (temporal bone resection excluding the ear, parotid gland removal, and neck dissection) with consideration of adjunctive radiotherapy.

Inner Ear Pathologies Causing CHL or MHL

Congenital or acquired pathologies of the inner ear can also be the cause of a CHL or MHL with ABG. These include semicircular canal dehiscence (abnormal thinning or loss of the temporal bone surrounding the canal), labyrinthine gushers, enlarged vestibular aqueduct, Mondini syndrome, Meniere's disease, and hydropic ear disease. In these cases, hearing loss is often mixed but can also be purely conductive. It is essential to identify all anomalies as they are differential diagnoses of middle ear pathologies such as otosclerosis. When missed out and surgery is performed, serious complications can arise including complete hearing loss. A thorough preoperative work-up with audiologic and vestibular examinations and imaging (CT or MRI) can identify these anomalies and avoid serious complications. Auditory rehabilitation ranges from standard HA to cochlear implants.

Conclusion

Conductive hearing loss and mixed hearing loss are often due to a defect of sound wave transmission in the external or middle ear, and in some cases the inner ear can be involved. Current examination tools (otoscopy, audio vestibular examination, imaging techniques) can offer precise diagnosis and management adapted to each patient's case surveillance, ossicular chain reconstruction, and tympanic membrane surgery, implantable and non-implantable HA.

References

1. Mittal R, Lisi CV, Gerring R, *et al.* (2015) Current concepts in the pathogenesis and treatment of chronic suppurative otitis media. *J Med Microbiol* **64**(10):1103–16.
2. Simon F, Haggard M, Rosenfeld RM, *et al.* (2018) International consensus (ICON) on management of otitis media with effusion in children. *Eur Ann Otorhinolaryngol Head Neck Dis* **135**(1S):S33–9.
3. Williams MT, Ayache D. (2006) Imaging in adult chronic otitis. *J Radiol* **87**(11 Pt 2):1743–55.
4. Schilder AGM, Marom T, Bhutta MF, *et al.* (2017) Panel 7: otitis media: Treatment and complications. *Otolaryngol Head Neck Surg* **156**(4_suppl):S88–105.
5. van Stekelenburg BCA, Aarts MCJ. (2019) Determinants influencing success rates of myringoplasty in daily practice: A retrospective analysis. *Eur Arch Otorhinolaryngol* **276**(11):3081–7.
6. McGee M, Hough JV. (1999) Ossiculoplasty. *Otolaryngol Clin North Am* **32**(3):471–88.
7. Ayache D, Schmerber S, Lavieille JP, *et al.* (2006) Middle ear cholesteatoma. *Ann Otolaryngol Chir Cervico* **123**(3):120–37.
8. Ayache D, Darrouzet V, Dubrulle F, *et al.* (2012) Imaging of non-operated cholesteatoma: Clinical practice guidelines. *Eur Ann Otorhinolaryngol Head Neck Dis* **129**(3):148–52.

9. Li B, Zhou L, Wang M, *et al.* (2021) Endoscopic versus microscopic surgery for treatment of middle ear cholesteatoma: A systematic review and meta-analysis. *Am J Otolaryngol* **42**(2):102451.
10. Daval M, Ayache D. (2018) Reconstruction of the canal wall in CWU tympanoplasty for cholesteatoma with titanium sheeting. *Otol Neurotol* **39**(2):258.
11. Ayache D, Manac'h F, Teszler CB, *et al.* (2017) Cartilage ossiculoplasty from stapes to tympanic membrane in one-stage intact canal wall tympanoplasty for cholesteatoma. *J Int Adv Otol* **13**(2):171–5.
12. Kerckhoffs KGP, Kommer MBJ, van Strien THL, *et al.* (2016) The disease recurrence rate after the canal wall up or canal wall down technique in adults. *Laryngoscope* **126**(4):980–7.
13. Saxby AJ, Jufas N, Kong JHK, *et al.* (2021) Novel radiologic approaches for cholesteatoma detection: Implications for endoscopic ear surgery. *Otolaryngol Clin North Am* **54**(1):89–109.
14. Williams MT, Ayache D. (2004) Imaging of the postoperative middle ear. *Eur Radiol* **14**(3):482–95.
15. Quesnel AM, Ishai R, McKenna MJ. (2018) Otosclerosis: Temporal bone pathology. *Otolaryngol Clin North Am* **51**(2):291–303.
16. Wolfovitz A, Luntz M. (2018) Impact of imaging in management of otosclerosis. *Otolaryngol Clin North Am* **51**(2):343–55.
17. Nguyen Y, Bernardeschi D, Sterkers O. (2018) Potential of robot-based surgery for otosclerosis surgery. *Otolaryngol Clin North Am* **51**(2):475–85.
18. Eshraghi AA, Ila K, Ocak E, Telischi FF. (2018) Advanced otosclerosis: Stapes surgery or cochlear implantation? *Otolaryngol Clin North Am* **51**(2):429–40.
19. Blanchard M, Abergel A, Vérillaud B, *et al.* (2011) Isolated malleus-handle fracture. *Auris Nasus Larynx* **38**(4):439–43.
20. Zhang TY, Bulstrode N, Chang KW, *et al.* (2019) International consensus recommendations on microtia, aural atresia and functional ear reconstruction. *J Int Adv Otol* **15**(2):204–8.

6 Current Medical Treatments for Sensorineural Hearing Loss

Sujana S. Chandrasekhar, MD, FACS[1–5]

Abstract

Sensorineural hearing loss (SNHL) is a symptom that may reflect a myriad of causes, and combines both cochlear ('sensory') and neural (nerve and/or brain) potential sites of lesion or injury. Therefore, there are several possible medical treatments for SNHL, and they are as targeted as possible to potential pathophysiological states. In this chapter, SNHL has been categorized as we often think of the clinical presentations, with treatments discussed for each, including presbycusis, noise-related hearing loss, fluctuating hearing loss, and sudden SNHL. As we learn more about correlations between untreated hearing loss and depression, isolation, and even dementia, it becomes all the more important to treat patients as best as possible to reverse the hearing loss. The reader should also keep in mind that hearing aid technology is an important part of our armamentarium and patients should be encouraged in their use if there is inadequate hearing recovery.

Overview

Sensorineural hearing loss (SNHL) is the most common type of hearing loss. The World Health Organization estimates that by the year 2050, nearly 2.5 billion of the projected 9.7 billion people in the world will have some degree of hearing loss and at least 700 million people will need some form of hearing rehabilitation.[1] Current medical treatments for SNHL focus on

Corresponding Author: Sujana S. Chandrasekhar, MD, FACS

[1] Cooperman Barnabas Medical Center, Livingston, NJ

[2] James J. Peters VA Medical Center, The Bronx, NY

[3] Lenox Hill Hospital (Northwell), New York, NY

[4] Manhattan Eye Ear and Throat Hospital (Northwell), New York, NY

[5] New York Eye And Ear Infirmary of Mt. Sinai, Mount Sinai Hospital, New York, NY

reversing it and preventing progression. Since tinnitus often accompanies SNHL, interventions including medications used to address the hearing loss often will help reduce the tinnitus as well.

As has been detailed earlier in this textbook, there are several pathophysiological mechanisms that can result in inner ear damage and thereby hearing loss. These include: structural abnormality of the cochlea and its components, usually congenital or traumatic in nature; aberrant metabolic activity that interferes with ion transport in the cochlea; interference with cochlear vascular supply, which can be as a result of various insults including noise trauma, ototoxicity, and systemic vascular events, all of which can affect the function of the stria vascularis; overcrowding of the basilar membrane with secondary reduction in outer hair cell (OHC) motility and inner hair cell transduction, which is prevalent in diabetes and autoimmune pathology; increase in vibrational shift between the tectorial and basilar membrane with secondary OHC stereocilia damage and increased stiffness of the organ of Corti, seen after noise trauma; and prevention of hair cell depolarization and change in perilymph ion concentration, as seen with aminoglycoside ototoxicity.[2]

Any treatments to prevent, treat, or prevent progression of hearing loss are therefore targeted to one or more of the mechanisms listed above.

Presbycusic SNHL

Presbycusis, or hearing loss of old age, usually begins in men in their 50s and women in their 60s and progresses slowly over time. Rarely does this go to the level of profound SNHL. At this time, we do not have medications that specifically treat progressive SNHL to reverse it or stop progression. We do, however, appreciate the interaction of systemic metabolic conditions, including hypercholesterolemia, hypertriglyceridemia, and impaired glucose metabolism with progression of presbycusic hearing loss.[3] Hyperlipidemia has independently been associated with tinnitus. In laboratory mice with diet-induced dyslipidemia, treatment with a statin prevented hearing impairment.[4] This type of data have not been generated for humans as of yet.

There is evidence that diabetes is associated with higher incidence and degree of presbycusis at all frequencies but specifically at the higher ones. The longer the duration of diabetes and the poorer the hemoglobin A1C control, the more severe the hearing loss is likely to be. The same is true for poorer control of hemoglobin A1C. Other evidence implies that the difference in hearing is not sustained between diabetics and non-diabetics over age 60. A population-based study found that Type 2 (non-insulin-dependent) diabetes was associated with prevalent, but not incident hearing loss in this older population. However, accelerated hearing loss progression over 5 years was more than doubled in persons newly diagnosed with diabetes.[5,6]

Cardiovascular diseases, smoking, and consumption of alcohol have often been mentioned as risk factors for presbycusis as well. In a large population-based study, smokers were 1.7 times as likely to have hearing loss as were non-smokers and the odds of having a hearing loss increased with pack-years of smoking and were higher for nonsmokers living with a current smoker.[7] The Framingham heart study, however, did not find such an association between hearing loss and smoking.[8]

The gut–brain axis has been widely studied, and gut dysbiosis, or imbalance in gut microbiome, serves as a predisposing factor for several neurological disorders including Alzheimer's disease, Parkinson's disease, multiple sclerosis, depression, anxiety, and autism spectrum disorder. The possibility of a gut–inner ear axis is suggested by: (1) autoimmune inner ear disease (AIED) when seen with other autoimmune disorders; (2) SNHL being the most common inner ear disorder that correlates with inflammatory bowel diseases; and (3) chronic noise exposure affecting the composition of gut microbiota and gastrointestinal tract inflammation.[9] Understanding this possibility and the need for ongoing research, it is still reasonable for otolaryngology physicians to counsel patients regarding healthy eating.

Physicians should advise patients to maintain optimal medical condition, which includes a healthy lifestyle avoiding risk factors as listed above. Control of real or nascent hyperlipidemia and diabetes control are encouraged, as well as avoidance of primary and secondary cigarette smoke exposure.

Noise-Induced Hearing Loss

In the United States, about 40 million people aged 20–69 years, and up to 17% of US adolescents have audiologic evidence of noise-induced hearing loss (NIHL) in one or both ears. The World Health Organization reports that 1.1 billion young people are at risk of NIHL. In middle- and high-income countries, 50% of young people listen to unsafe levels of sound through personal audio devices; 40% are exposed to damaging sound at entertainment venues. In 2022, the WHO released a new global standard for safe listening venues and events.[10] Level of noise exposure needed to experience damage is as little as 5 hours per week of exposure to sound over 85 dB in intensity.

Understanding of NIHL has expanded to appreciate that impulse noises and continuous noises can lead to NIHL. Classically, temporary threshold shifts (TTSs) are considered reversible and recoverable while repeated TTS eventually results in permanent threshold shift (PTS). The epicenter of cochlear hair cell damage and nerve fiber degeneration in NIHL is at the cochlear region that corresponds to the 4 kHz response area. A 'noise notch' centered at 4 kHz is the earliest sign; with continued noise exposure and damage, the 'V' of the notch extends, more towards the basilar turn (higher frequencies are encompassed in the loss) and eventually to involve the apical (lower) frequencies as noise exposure persists. The degree of hearing loss from noise can reach up to 70–90 dB. There are animal data supporting the concept that even mild acoustic trauma can result in the loss of more than 50% of synapses between cochlear nerve fibers. This is postulated to cause 'hidden hearing loss,' in which we cannot measure threshold degradation but the patient reports difficulty hearing, particularly in background or competing noise situations.[11] More data are needed to verify the clinical validity of cochlear synaptopathy, diagnostic measures, and possible treatments.

Obviously, prevention is the best treatment. Noise avoidance and regular use of personal protective hearing equipment is the standard of care. Governmental standards for industrial controls have been in place in many countries. Still, NIHL remains the most preventable cause of permanent hearing loss around the world.

There are no pharmaceutical compounds shown to prevent, treat, or reverse NIHL at this time. Experimental animal studies with systemic or local antioxidants have shown both hair cell protection and reduction of NIHL. N-acetyl cysteine (NAC) is unusual in that it has been studied in both animal and human trials, for NIHL. NAC replenishes cysteine which allows for glutathione (GSH) synthesis. Glutathione is a major antioxidant enzyme in inner ear hair cells. NAC in and of itself also acts as a scavenger of reactive oxygen species (ROS). The data are compelling in animal studies, with both inner hair cell and OHC loss reduction as well as reduced auditory brainstem response and otoacoustic emission shifts in treated animals. Results have varied in humans. The largest such trial to date was conducted by the US Department of the Navy in which 566 Marine Corps subjects received 900 mg of either NAC or placebo with each meal (total 2,700 mg/day) during the first 16 days of weapon training. Significant decreases in threshold shift rates were seen when handedness was considered.[12] Other studies have shown mixed results. NAC's role as a reliable otoprotectant in NIHL remains to be firmly established.

Other antioxidants studied in animals but not in humans include methionine, acetyl-l-carnitine, and Resveratrol. Studies of these and other agents are needed, as well as an understanding of the value of pre- versus post-treatment, and how long treatment may be delayed after noise exposure but still remain effective.

Fluctuating SNHL

Meniere's disease (MD), whose pathological correlate is endolymphatic hydrops, and autoimmune ear disease (AIED) are both associated with fluctuations in sensorineural hearing. This is most often in the lower frequencies but not so limited. Cochlear hydrops is a subset of MD where the patient gives a history of fluctuating aural fullness, tinnitus, and hearing loss without vertigo or vestibular symptoms. This entity was excluded by the Committee on Hearing and Equilibrium of the American Academy of Otolaryngology-Head and Neck Surgery (AAO-HNS) in 1985 but more recent radiologic imaging studies seem to demonstrate this pathological condition.[13] Once the diagnosis of either MD or AIED has been made, counselling relates to dietary management and medical treatment as first-line interventions.

Meniere's Disease

As per the European Position Statement on MD,[14] a personalized approach for MD patients is strongly recommended. Therefore, treating a presenting comorbid condition such as allergy, migraine, or autoimmune arthritis is important. Although there is no currently available gene therapy for this disorder, it is recommended that the clinician obtain appropriate familial history of hearing loss and episodes of vertigo. Genetic testing will identify the causal variant in 30% of familial cases, paving the way for gene therapy in few years.

In the United States, sodium restriction is the norm for patients with MD. The AAO-HNS Clinical Practice Guideline (CPG) on MD[15] details the relatively low evidence basis, but found enough evidence to recommend a low-sodium diet, between 1,500 and 2,300 mg of sodium per day. This is from the American Heart Association's recommendation for a heart-healthy diet. Studies show that sodium may induce an increase in the plasma aldosterone concentration that can activate ion transport and absorption of endolymph in the endolymphatic sac.

There is no evidence supporting other dietary restrictions that are commonly discussed with patients, including restriction of caffeine, nicotine, and alcohol. However, after these possibilities are discussed with the patient, they may identify a beneficial effect to themselves with these types of consumption modifications. Likewise, there are no data for or against the use of cannabinoids in treating patients with MD.

An association between allergy and MD has been shown in cross-sectional and observational studies, while animal studies have shown evidence of allergic activity within the inner ear. There are no randomized controlled trials regarding allergy testing and treatment in relation to reducing the symptoms of MD. However, there are ample other types of studies demonstrating significant benefit for vertigo, hearing loss, and tinnitus in patients with MD and allergies who receive allergy treatment. Given the low risk to patients, inclusion of allergen avoidance and immunotherapy should be considered in the treatment plan to help patients control MD symptoms. Again, personalized care is important here. The clinician should ask the patient if they experience changes in their MD symptoms with seasonal or other allergies and/or with changes in barometric pressure. Treatment with antihistamines may afford great benefit in susceptible individuals.

Diuretics and betahistine are used in MD for symptom control, primarily for vertigo but may also be beneficial for hearing loss/ear fullness and tinnitus. Diuretics are believed to alter the electrolyte balance in endolymph, subsequently reducing endolymph volume. The most commonly used ones for MD are once-daily thiazides with or without potassium-sparing diuretics such as hydrochlorothiazide/triamterene or spironolactone or the carbonic anhydrase inhibitor acetazolamide, which is given twice daily as a second-line therapy. Betahistine dihydrochloride is a histamine analogue that strongly antagonized histamine H3 receptors and acts as a weak agonist on histamine H1 receptors. The recommended dosage for MD is 16 mg thrice daily with meals. The data for vertigo are relatively weak and are even more so for pure hearing loss. The AAO-HNS CPG[15] states that these medications are an option for MD. The clinician should bear in mind that an individual patient may, in fact, respond to these interventions, and should act accordingly.

Oral antiviral treatments may control the cochlear and/or vestibular symptoms of MD. One small study showed nearly 40% hearing improvement after 3 weeks of thrice-daily dosage, 3 weeks of twice-daily dosage, and 1 year of once-daily antiviral.[16] A short course of oral steroid therapy is unlikely to improve hearing in MD, based on a few small studies. A histological study in guinea pigs showed dilation of the endolymphatic space in the animals given glucocorticoids, which is the opposite of the effect we are trying to achieve when treating humans who have MD with steroids. Intratympanic (IT) steroids are also listed as an option for the treatment of MD in the AAO-HNS CPG. Most studies on this modality discuss vertigo control and not cochlear symptoms. One study indicates that IT steroids are effective for vertigo control but not for hearing loss and tinnitus. Another suggests that IT steroids improve quality of life (QOL) in MD, in the domains of vertigo and instability, but not for hearing, tinnitus, or aural fullness. However, the personalized treatment plan of the patient at hand may include some or all of the above-mentioned treatments, if they control their symptoms.

Autoimmune Ear Disease

A key feature of AIED is improved hearing as a response to immunosuppressive therapy — corticosteroids. Unless there are medical contraindications, aggressive, long-term treatment with systemic steroids should be considered. Short-term bursts of steroids are insufficient and may result in relapse. Although regimens are not standardized, many recommend prednisone 1 mg/kg/day for 1 month followed by a slow taper over several weeks to reach a maintenance dose of 10–20 mg/day where the hearing is stable. Occasional increases in doses are needed as the AIED activity increases and hearing drops. Overall steroid response rates are 60% and are defined as improvement in hearing of 15 dB at one frequency, 10 dB at two consecutive frequencies, or a significant improvement in word discrimination score. Long-term steroid use is not without risk and this treatment calls for significant shared decision-making.[17]

Cytotoxic medications are used for people who are steroid-intolerant or in whom their hearing fails to demonstrate a continued response to steroids. Potential adverse effects of the cytotoxic medication must be discussed, as they are potentially serious. For example, risks of cyclophosphamide include myelosuppression, hemorrhagic cystitis, infertility, and increased risk of malignancy. Other agents that have been used for AIED include methotrexate (MTX) and azathioprine (trade name: Imuran®). Later studies showed that MTX was not better than high-dose prednisone. More recently, etanercept (trade name: Enbrel®) has been tried and although hearing improvement was not seen, hearing stabilization of previously progressive SNHL was shown.

N-acetyl cysteine has previously been discussed regarding NIHL. It is an antioxidant that also discourages the lipopolysaccharide-mediated release of tumor necrosis factor alpha (TNF-α) from peripheral blood mononuclear cells in patients with AIED while only minimally affecting the same pathway's downstream targets.[18] The interleukin (IL)-1 receptor antagonist anakinra was studied in corticosteroid-resistant AIED patients in a small Phase I/II study of 10 patients and showed improvement in 7 patients with relapse in 3 after therapy was discontinued. A Phase II study is underway.

Sudden SNHL

Sudden hearing loss is a frightening symptom that is frequently, but not universally, accompanied by tinnitus and/or vertigo. Sudden sensorineural hearing loss (SSNHL) affects 5–27 per 100,000 people annually, with about 66,000 new cases per year in the United States. There are a number of options for treatment, but the current understanding is that the earlier that treatment is instituted, the better the likelihood of hearing recovery is.[19]

The International Consensus on SSNHL points out the heterogeneity of causes of the symptom SSNHL that confound interpretation of treatment outcomes.[20]

As a rule, but of course not universally, mild-to-moderate SSNHL, especially that affecting low or mid frequencies, tends to recover, while severe-to-profound SSNHL, and high-frequency SNHL, tends not to recover. The concept of the mid-audiogram 'steroid effective zone' was introduced in 1980 and holds true today. In moderate-to-severe mid-frequency SSNHL, steroids offer over 4:1 increased odds of hearing recovery. There is a strong role for shared decision-making when offering observation or treatment for SSNHL. The author's personal approach is one of aggressive treatment to maximize the chance of recovery of this most important sense.

Systemic Steroids

Prednisone 1 mg/kg for 7–10 days followed by a taper, or the equivalent of another systemic steroid, is an option per the AAO-HNS/F CPGs[21] if given within 2 weeks of onset. However, it is understood that many patients do not present in that time frame, and those who present after 2 weeks, have passed the window of expected spontaneous recovery. Many neurotologists, therefore, continue to offer this first-line type of systemic steroid treatment to patients within the first 6–8 weeks of onset.

Intratympanic Steroids

The AAO-HNS/F CPG states that IT steroids are an option in primary treatment within 2 weeks of onset and recommends IT steroids for salvage therapy in patients whose onset of SSNHL was 2–6 weeks prior. Dexamethasone and methylprednisolone are the commonly used agents. As methylprednisolone may cause a burning sensation in the middle ear, dexamethasone appears to be more commonly used. There are numerous articles evaluating dexamethasone 4 or 5 mg/ml, but higher concentrations appear to show better outcomes. It is this author's experience and noted in a small retrospective study of 37 patients[22] that dexamethasone 24 mg/ml delivered intratympanically is superior to dexamethasone 10 mg/ml. Injections are commonly delivered every 3–7 days for a total of 3 or 4, or until hearing is restored. The injection technique is detailed in the AAO-HNS/F CPG. Facilitators of round window transport such as histamine and hyaluronic acid have been studied[23] but are not commercially available.

Systemic vs. Intratympanic Steroids

Studies have shown that neither form of steroid delivery is superior. Combination of both may prove to be superior, particularly in severe-to-profound SSNHL. Adverse drug reactions are more pronounced in systemic treatment.[24,25]

Hyperbaric Oxygen

Although increasing in use, the published data only support HBOT as an option *if combined with steroid therapy* in the initial management of SSNHL within 2 weeks or as salvage within 1 month of onset.[21,25]

Other Pharmacologic Therapy

The AAO-HNS/F CPG strongly recommends against the routine prescription of antivirals, thrombolytics, vasodilators, or vasoactive substances to patients with SSNHL.[21] However, this does not preclude the use of clinical judgment in personalizing healthcare.

Summary

Helen Keller, who had both hearing and vision impairment, famously said, 'Blindness cuts us off from things, but deafness cuts us off from people.' It is an honor and a privilege to have the education and expertise to help our patients when they confront the frightening prospect of losing such an important sense as their hearing. I encourage all of us to continue to care for and listen to our patients, learn from them, and learn from all of the research that is ongoing and will happen, to do all that we can to help them achieve the outcomes they are seeking.

References

1. World Health Organization. (2021) *Deafness and Hearing Loss*. https://www.who.int/news-room/fact-sheets/detail/deafness-and-hearing-loss
2. Tanna RJ, Lin JW, De Jesus O. (2022) *Sensorineural Hearing Loss*. [Updated 2022 May 15]. In: StatPearls [Internet]. Treasure Island, FL: StatPearls Publishing. Available from https://www.ncbi.nlm.nih.gov/books/NBK565860/.
3. Evans MB, Tonini R, Shope CD, *et al.* (2006) Dyslipidemia and auditory function. *Otol Neurotol* **27**(5):609–14. doi:10.1097/01.mao.0000226286.19295.34. PMID: 16868509; PMCID: PMC3607507.
4. Lee YY, Choo O-S, Kim YJ, *et al.* (2020) Atorvastatin prevents hearing impairment in the presence of hyperlipidemia. *Biochim Biophys Acta Mol Cell Res* **1867**(12):118850.
5. Vaughan N, James K, McDermott D, *et al.* (2006) A 5-year prospective study of diabetes and hearing loss in a veteran population. *Otol Neurotol* **27**(1):37–43. doi:10.1097/01.mao.0000194812.69556.74.
6. Mitchell P, Gopinath B, McMahon CM, *et al.* (2009) Relationship of type 2 diabetes to the prevalence, incidence and progression of age-related hearing loss. *Diabetic Med* **26**(5):483–8. doi:10.1111/j.1464-5491.2009.02710.x.
7. Cruickshanks KJ, Klein R, Klein BEK, *et al.* (1998) Cigarette smoking and hearing loss: The epidemiology of hearing loss study. *JAMA* **279**(21):1715–9. doi:10.1001/jama.279.21.1715.
8. Gates GA, Cobb JL, D'Agostino RB, Wolf PA. (1993) The relation of hearing in the elderly to the presence of cardiovascular disease and cardiovascular risk factors. *Arch Otolaryngol Head Neck Surg* **119**:156–61.
9. Denton AJ, Godur DA, Mittal J, *et al.* (2022) Recent advancements in understanding the gut microbiome and the inner ear axis. *Otolaryngol Clin North Am* **55**(5):1125–37. doi:10.1016/j.otc.2022.07.002.
10. World Health Organization. (2022) *WHO Global Standard for Safe Listening Venues and Events*. World Health Organization, viii, 107 p. https://apps.who.int/iris/handle/10665/352277. Accessed Oct 23, 2022.
11. Liberman MC. (2016) Noise-induced hearing loss: Permanent versus temporary threshold shifts and the effects of hair cell versus neuronal degeneration. *Adv Exp Med Biol* **875**:1–7.
12. Kopke R, Slade MD, Jackson R, *et al.* (2015) Efficacy and safety of N-acetylcysteine in prevention of noise induced hearing loss: A randomized clinical trial. *Hear Res* **323**:40–50.
13. Alonso JE, Ishiyama GP, Fujiwara RJT, *et al.* (2021) Cochlear Meniere's: A distinct clinical entity with isolate cochlear hydrops on high-resolution MRI? *Front Surg* **8**:680260.

14. Magnan J, Özgirgin ON, Trabalzini F, *et al.* (2018) European position statement on diagnosis, and treatment of Meniere's disease. *J Int Adv Otol* **14**(2):317–21. doi:10.5152/iao.2018.140818. PMID: 30256205; PMCID: PMC6354459.
15. Basura GJ, Adams ME, Monfared A, *et al.* (2020) Clinical practice guideline: Meniere's disease. *Otolaryngol Head Neck Surg* **162**(2 Suppl):S1–55.
16. Gacek RR. (2015) Recovery of hearing in Meniere's disease after antiviral treatment. *Am J Otolaryngol* **36**(3):315–23. doi:10.1016/j.amjoto.2014.03.016. Epub 2014 Apr 5. PMID: 25940200.
17. Vambutas A, Pathak S. (2016) AAO: Autoimmune and autoinflammatory (disease) in otology: What is new in immune-mediated hearing loss. *Laryngoscope Investig Otolaryngol* **1**(5):110–5.
18. Pathak S, Stern C, Vambutas A. (2015) *N*-acetylcysteine attenuates tumor necrosis factor alpha levels in autoimmune inner ear disease patients. *Immunol Res* **63**(1–3):236–45.
19. Chandrasekhar SS, Tsai Do BS, Schwartz SR, *et al.* (2019) Clinical practice guideline: Sudden hearing loss (update) executive summary. *Otolaryngol Head Neck Surg* **161**(2):195–210.
20. Marx M, Younes E, Chandrasekhar SS, *et al.* (2018) International consensus (ICON) on treatment of sudden sensorineural hearing loss. *Eur Ann Otorhinolaryngol Head Neck Dis* **135**(1 Suppl):S23–8.
21. Alexander TH, Harris JP, Nguyen QT, Vorasubin N. (2015) Dose effect of intratympanic dexamethasone for idiopathic sudden sensorineural hearing loss: 24 mg/mL is superior to 10 mg/mL. *Otol Neurotol* **36**(8):1321–7.
22. Chandrasekhar SS, Rubinstein RY, Kwartler JA, *et al.* (2000) Dexamethasone pharmacokinetics in the inner ear: Comparison of route of administration and use of facilitating agents. *Otolaryngol Head Neck Surg* **122**:521–8.
23. Mirian C, Ovesen T. (2020) Intratympanic vs systemic corticosteroids in first-line treatment of idiopathic sudden sensorineural hearing loss: A systematic review and meta-analysis. *JAMA Otolaryngol Head Neck Surg* **146**(5):421–8.
24. Rauch SD, Halpin CF, Antonelli PJ, *et al.* (2011) Oral vs intratympanic corticosteroid therapy for idiopathic sudden sensorineural hearing loss: A randomized trial. *JAMA* **305**(20):2071–9.
25. Rhee T, Hwang D, Lee J, *et al.* (2018) Addition of hyperbaric oxygen therapy vs medical therapy alone for idiopathic sudden sensorineural hearing loss: A systematic review and meta-analysis. *JAMA Otolaryngol Head Neck Surg* **144**(12):1153–61.

7 Assessment and Management of Tinnitus and Hyperacusis

Ali A. Danesh, PhD[1]; Ava King, BSc[2]; Adrien A. Eshraghi, MD, MSc, FACS[2]

Abstract

Tinnitus is a sound that is usually perceived within the head or ears. The current available health data suggest that roughly 10% of the US population have experienced tinnitus that lasts at least 5 minutes. Typically, a tinnitus that lasts <5 minutes is not considered as pathologic or significant. Tinnitus does not have any external source and it can be described as ringing, roaring, and static sounds or it may be perceived like a pulse. Tinnitus has been categorized as primary or secondary tinnitus. Primary tinnitus is usually associated with sensorineural hearing loss and the secondary tinnitus is frequently accompanied by other conditions such as ear infections or cardiovascular issues. Tinnitus is a pathologically heterogeneous ailment. This means that a variety of conditions can be associated with tinnitus or cause tinnitus. Tinnitus is a manageable condition and there are a variety of effective methods that are used in tinnitus centers around the world to help those who suffer from it. Providing empathic care and support to the patient from the clinician's side and motivation and determination in getting better from the patient's side usually result in significant reduction in the annoyance caused by tinnitus. Addressing the factors of sensation, emotion, and cognition in the management of tinnitus is essential. When tinnitus is associated with hearing loss, specific medical or surgical approach may also be used in parallel to sound or cognitive therapies.

Corresponding author: Ali A. Danesh, PhD

[1] Department of Communication Sciences and Disorders and Integrated Medical Sciences Schmidt College of Medicine, Florida Atlantic University, Boca Raton, FL, United States.

[2] Hearing Research and Cochlear Implant Laboratory, University of Miami, Miami, FL, United States.

Tinnitus Diagnosis, Evaluations, and Causes

Tinnitus: Definition and History

For thousands of years people have suffered from tinnitus and it has been a great challenge for many of the medical professionals to find a way to cure it. The word *tinnitus* comes from the Latin word *tinnire*, which means to ring or tinkle. Tinnitus is a sound that is usually perceived within the head or ears. Tinnitus does not have any external source and it can be described as ringing, roaring, static sounds or it may sound like a pulse. There are many references to *tinnitus* throughout the history of medicine, including the report of the papyri from Ancient Egypt about tinnitus, which has been considered as controversial by some[1]; however, the works of Persian medical scholars of the middle ages such as Avicenna[2] and the efforts of the French otologist Jean Marc Gaspard Itard[3] are notable.

Classification of Tinnitus

Most of the medical community categorizes tinnitus into subjective and objective classes. A subjective tinnitus is the most common type, which can be heard only by the individuals with tinnitus. On the contrary, an objective tinnitus is a sound that can be heard not only by the patient, but can also be detected or heard by others. Most recently, tinnitus has been labelled as **primary or secondary.**[4] Primary tinnitus is usually associated with sensorineural hearing loss and the secondary tinnitus is accompanied by other conditions such as middle ear fluid, Eustachian tube malfunction, abnormal blood flow or vascular disease and therefore it has a specific and known reason. Tinnitus can be acute or chronic, with acute tinnitus lasting less than three months and chronic tinnitus lasting more than three months. Not all of the tinnitus complaints can be bothersome. Tinnitus for some individuals can be intermittent or constant and it may interfere with their sleep or concentration. Tinnitus can cause emotional reactions, fear, difficulty in relaxation or clear thinking. There are millions of individuals who have perceived tinnitus with no annoyance. One can address them as '*a person with tinnitus*' rather than '*a tinnitus patient*' who significantly is annoyed by it! Tinnitus can vary in loudness. It can be soft for some or loud to others. It can be a high-pitched or a low-pitched sound; it can be heard in the head or in the ears, one ear or both. Transient sounds such as hearing a few seconds of ringing is not usually referred to as tinnitus and considered as a spontaneous activity of the auditory system.

Prevalence of Tinnitus

Tinnitus has been coined as the malady of the 21st century. The increase in noise pollution, advancing age, and use of medications have contributed to the augmented prevalence of tinnitus. The American Tinnitus Association has estimated that around 50 million people in the USA have tinnitus. This may include people who have heard tinnitus temporarily. Usually, a tinnitus that lasts <5 minutes is not considered as pathologic or significant. The data from the National Center for Health Statistics from the Center for Disease Control and Prevention and reports from the National Institute of Deafness and other Communication Disorders suggest that roughly 10% of the population in the US have experienced tinnitus that lasts at least 5 minutes. Globally speaking, we can estimate that around 700 million people in our planet have tinnitus, which is roughly 10% of the Earth's population. However, of these, about 50% of patients with tinnitus have seen a healthcare provider, and 8% have severe tinnitus.

What Causes Tinnitus?

Tinnitus is a pathologically heterogeneous ailment. This means that a variety of conditions can be associated with tinnitus or cause tinnitus. Tinnitus can be a sign of a benign condition or it may be due to more complicated diseases. There is not much evidence for a genetic cause of tinnitus. There are some gene candidates such as RCOR1, a neuronal repressor; however, a hereditary trait has not been identified yet.[5] No matter which underlying condition causes tinnitus, it usually can be managed. Here we will examine the basis for tinnitus and what causes its generation.

Subjective tinnitus, the type that is heard only by the patient, is the most common class of tinnitus. Noise exposure including an acoustic trauma is the major cause of subjective tinnitus. Noise exposure can damage the structures within the cochlea and destroy the delicate sensory cells inside the inner ear. This in turn causes a hearing impairment, which is called sensorineural hearing loss. This loss of hair cells is the major reason of sensorineural hearing losses, which may originate from aging, medications, or noise exposure. Unlike other species such as fish, birds, and sharks;

mammals, including humans of course, cannot replace or regenerate these delicate hair cells and damage to the hair cells is permanent. It is believed that some of the reasons for subjective tinnitus is due to the underlying sensorineural hearing loss. Researchers believe that the lack of message transmission from the ear to the brain results in changes in the auditory centers, particularly in the auditory cortex, which produces tinnitus. This phenomenon is comparable to the concept of phantom limb. Many amputated individuals who have lost one or more of their extremities such as arms and legs may complain about a phantom sensation or phantom pain from an organ that is non-existing. The explanation about this phenomenon is very likely related to the changes in our somatosensory cortex on the parietal lobe of our brain. It is believed that the areas of the parietal cortex that are responsible for the sensation from a leg or an arm are being used by other parts of the body, hence generating a sensation of the missing organ. This analogy has been applied in the auditory neuroscience. If the brain cannot 'hear' signals, it will make a phantom auditory sensation, which we call tinnitus and it is believed to be due to neuroplasticity (i.e., changes in the neural pathways).[7] Although the concept of neuroplasticity about tinnitus is very attractive, it does not explain why millions of people with significant hearing loss do not have tinnitus and why there are many patients with tinnitus with essentially normal hearing thresholds. In addition to the noise exposure, tinnitus and sensorineural hearing loss can be due to the use of ototoxic (poisonous to the ear) medications. The ototoxic medications include a variety of aminoglycoside antibiotics, antimalarial, and anticancer drugs.

A variety of other conditions cause subjective tinnitus. A skilled clinician will start with a thorough inspection of the ear canal and comprehensive hearing evaluation that includes tests of the middle ear, inner ear, the auditory nerve, and the rest of the auditory neural pathways. Sometimes cerumen or abnormalities of the ear canal is the underlying reason. Other contributing factors may be related to disorders of the temporomandibular joint (TMJ) or cervical abnormalities. Table 7.1 presents some of the reasons for subjective tinnitus and potential therapeutic approaches.

Objective tinnitus is the less common type of tinnitus. Patients with objective tinnitus may be significantly annoyed by the sound of their tinnitus and may report it as a pounding sound. An objective tinnitus may represent itself as a pulse (synchronous with the heartbeats) or may sound like a click (usually spasm of the muscles of the middle ear or the soft palate

Table 7.1 Some of the most common reasons of subjective tinnitus.

Origin of Tinnitus	External ear	Middle ear	Inner ear	Auditory nerve and beyond	Other organs or parts of the body
Etiology of Tinnitus	Impaction of cerumen Blockage of the ear canal	Otitis media Otosclerosis Abrupt pressure change (barotrauma) Ruptured or perforated tympanic membrane	Meniere's disease Acoustic trauma Ototoxic medications Aging Viral infections	Vestibular schwannoma/ acoustic neuroma Brain tumors Meningioma	Endocrinal disorders (diabetes, thyroid disease), Hormonal changes, Migraine, TMJ
What to do for it?	Remove cerumen and blockage	Otologic management (ie. antibiotic treatment, middle ear surgery...)	Otologic and audiologic management (ie. Meniere's diet, appropriate medications, hearing devices...)	Neurosurgical and neurotologic management (ie. watchful observation, radiosurgery, surgical removal...)	Internal medicine, endocrinology, neurology, and psychiatry, oral surgery

is the source). An objective tinnitus can be secondary to conditions such as benign intracranial hypertension, glomus jugulare tumor, arterial bruits, atherosclerosis of the carotid artery, transverse sinus stenosis, microvascular compression of the auditory-vestibular nerve, sigmoid sinus dehiscence, and other types of vascular or blood flow disorders. A Doppler ultrasound study of the carotid arteries, magnetic resonance angiography (MRA), magnetic resonance venography (MRV), or computed tomography angiography (CTA) of the head and neck are useful tools to study such disorders. The carotid Doppler ultrasound studies can show the diameter of the carotid artery and its diastolic velocity and help in the management of pulsatile tinnitus.

Tinnitus Assessment

The impact of tinnitus on the patient's life and daily activities is an important component of tinnitus assessment. There are many psychometrically validated questionnaires for tinnitus. The Tinnitus Handicap Inventory (THI)[8] and Tinnitus Functional Index[9] are two of the commonly used questionnaires. A newly developed questionnaire named Tinnitus Impact Questionnaire (Figure 7.1) is a useful tool that focuses on a variety of factors and assesses

Tinnitus Impact Questionnaire

Over the last 2 weeks, how often would you say the following has occurred because of hearing a sound in your ears or head with no external source (e.g., buzzing, a high-pitched whistle, hissing...)?				
1. Lack of concentration	0–1 day	2–6 days	7–10 days	11–14 days
2. Feeling anxious	0–1 day	2–6 days	7–10 days	11–14 days
3. Sleep difficulties (delay in falling asleep and/or difficulty getting back to sleep if woken up during the night)	0–1 night	2–6 nights	7–10 nights	11–14 nights
4. Lack of enjoyment from leisure activities	0–1 day	2–6 days	7–10 days	11–14 days
5. Inability to perform certain day-to-day activities/tasks	0–1 day	2–6 days	7–10 days	11–14 days
6. Feeling irritable	0–1 day	2–6 days	7–10 days	11–14 days
7. Low mood	0–1 day	2–6 days	7–10 days	11–14 days

Fig. 7.1 Tinnitus Impact Questionnaire measures the impact of tinnitus on a variety of factors influencing tinnitus (adopted from Aazh *et al.*).[10]

the impact of tinnitus on the patient's day-to-day activities, mood, and sleep, and not on hearing difficulties.[10] These tools can help in the determination of the level of annoyance from tinnitus from multiple dimensions such as concentration, sleep, relationships, and communication.

The evaluation for objective and pulsatile tinnitus usually starts with the inspection of the external auditory canals, evaluation of the middle ear function and Eustachian tube function, and examination of the muscles of the oral cavity. This may also be followed by the examination and checking the TMJ. Pulsatile tinnitus may be due to atherosclerosis (plaques in the arteries) of arteries close to the ear, particularly the internal carotid artery. A skilled clinician will explore the auscultation sounds from the head and neck for a single or multiple potential cause of an objective or pulsatile tinnitus. Imaging techniques such as carotid Doppler ultrasound evaluation, magnetic resonance imaging (MRI), MRA, or CT angiogram of the head and neck (temporal bones) are valuable tools that can provide more information in studying objective and pulsatile tinnitus.

For the assessment of the more commonly seen subjective tinnitus, which is heard only by the patient, a variety of the procedures are employed. We need to keep in mind that tinnitus is not a real sound and patients need to be aware that tinnitus is an electrochemical activity of the brain that is perceived as sounds. Although we cannot 'see' tinnitus, we can spot tinnitus-related activity with neuroimaging techniques. Many patients with tinnitus can 'evoke' their tinnitus or modify its loudness. This evoked tinnitus can be heard by the patient through the initiation of the movement of the eyes (i.e., gaze-evoked tinnitus) or by the movement of their jaw and limbs. With the use of neuroimaging techniques such as functional MRI and positron emission tomography[11] scientists have been able to detect and image tinnitus-related activity in a variety of brain structures, including brainstem (particularly midbrain), thalamus, and cortex.[12]

The assessment for tinnitus should include a comprehensive evaluation of hearing, middle ear, and the inner ear. Usually, pure-tone audiometry, speech audiometry, tympanometry, and otoacoustic emissions (a response from the cells within the inner ear) are fundamental and necessary tests. Following the comprehensive audiological evaluation, psychoacoustic tinnitus measurements are the next step. The psychoacoustic assessment includes tinnitus pitch match, tinnitus loudness match, tinnitus minimal masking level, and residual inhibition test. The evidence from tinnitus assessment procedures provides clinicians with the information that can help in better diagnosis, understanding, and treatment options.

Consequences of Tinnitus

Tinnitus by itself interferes with concentration, sleep, relaxation, social interactions and may be associated with or exacerbate underlying depression, insomnia, stress, fear, isolation, and anxiety. Tinnitus is not a psychiatric disorder nor a psychological condition. It is a real phenomenon that causes distress to the individual and can happen acutely in a short time after an impact noise exposure or use of ototoxic medications or it can be a persistent condition where it accumulates and increases over a longer period of time. An intermittent tinnitus that lasts for a few minutes occasionally does not usually distress the patient and a session of examination followed by counselling results in a good outcome. Tinnitus becomes an important issue when it is continuous and when it interferes with the daily activities or sleep patterns of the patient. Sometimes tinnitus can result in psychosomatic reactions such as feeling of pain in the ears, pressure in the ears, headaches, tenderness of the muscles of head and neck, and a feeling of being disoriented. All of these symptoms are usually a sign of psychologic burden of tinnitus and they are more controlled as the patient advances into the management stage.

Tinnitus Management

Depending on how we define cure, currently we have no *cure* for chronic tinnitus. If our definition of cure means that tinnitus will absolutely disappear following a therapeutic procedure, then it must be stated that at least for now no such method is available. In other words, our current knowledge and skills in tinnitus treatment does not eliminate tinnitus. However, if by cure we are referring to the ability to give a better control of tinnitus and reduce its associative symptoms, then we absolutely can tell our patients that tinnitus is curable, although, we prefer to use the term manageable. A significant number of the US population experience tinnitus and a lot of healthcare providers are dismissive about tinnitus and have unsympathetic attitude towards tinnitus patients. Healthcare providers need to know that a lot can be done for tinnitus patients that can reduce their discomfort from this ailment. Reassuring the patient by explaining to them that tinnitus is not a terminal disease or a dangerous and life-threatening disorder is useful in their journey to recovery. All clinicians should be aware that tinnitus is pretty much a manageable condition. There are several management methods for tinnitus and not all of them are approved approaches based on evidence and research. Therefore, more emphasis will be given to Evidence-Based Practice management strategies. However, some alternative or complementary methods of tinnitus management will be reviewed as well.

Useful clinical practice guidelines for tinnitus management have been provided by a group of clinical scientists that include recommendations for evaluation and assessment of the impact of tinnitus on individuals and identification of the efficacious interventions in the management of tinnitus and its weight on the quality of life of those who suffer from it.[13] According to the guidelines and the review of the studies, there are many protocols and methods for tinnitus management and for many of these methods there is not enough evidence of their effectiveness at this time. A list of tinnitus management methods may include the use of supplements, medications, electrical stimulations, repeated transcranial magnetic stimulation,[14] neuro-biofeedback, sound therapy, counselling, and cognitive behavioral therapy (CBT), just to name a few.

We will discuss various management options in this section. There are many methods that show some level of promise with evidence-based studies and are successful in alleviating persistent tinnitus and improving quality of life in individuals with annoying and bothersome persistent tinnitus. These include electrical stimulation, sound therapy (i.e., use of acoustical stimulations), and CBT. However, the next sections will explore various other approaches offered at this time to patients that may be used as a complementary approach by practitioners.

Electrical Stimulation

Use of electrical stimulation to alleviate a wide range of medical conditions is not new. For decades electrical stimulation has been used to reduce pain, treat psychiatric and neurologic disorders, or to improve the function of paralyzed organs. The application of deep brain stimulation (DBS) in specific parts of the brain in the management of conditions such as Parkinson's disease and severe cases of obsessive-compulsive disorders (OCD) has shown to be very effective. The idea of electrical stimulation for tinnitus suppression has been examined on different parts of the body, including electrodermal stimulation of the surface of the wrists, electrical stimulation of the ear canals, and most recently on the tongue.[15] The bimodal (electrical and auditory stimulations) has been shown to have neuromodulatory effects and to result in a significant reduction in tinnitus symptoms (Figure 7.2). The DBS approach may not be effective at this time for electrical suppression of tinnitus as we are not able to identify which part of the brain is generating

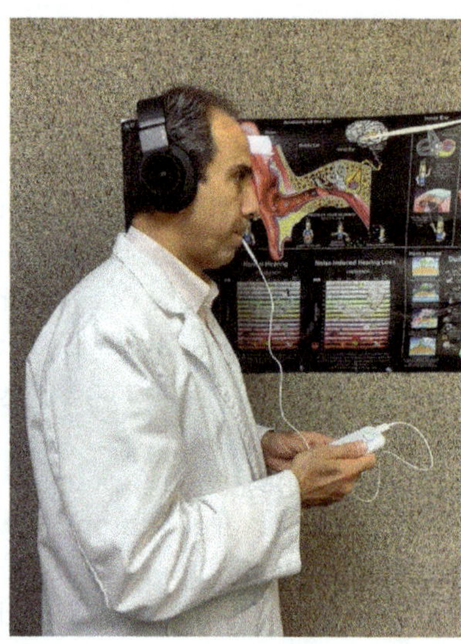

Fig. 7.2 Bimodal neuromodulation for tinnitus suppression by combining acoustic signals and electrical stimulation of the tongue (Linire, Ireland).

tinnitus in each affected patient. Electrical stimulation via the use of cochlear implants has been shown to be effective in individuals with severe to profound hearing loss and tinnitus. Patients report that while their cochlear implant device is ON, they do not hear their tinnitus; however, they perceive their tinnitus again when they remove their implants.

Sound Therapy

Sound therapy is another effective method in the management of tinnitus. Many tinnitus patients report that they do not hear their tinnitus in the presence of background noise or when they take a shower. It seems that the noise from such environments mixes with their tinnitus and reduces its volume. These kinds of reports from patients encouraged clinicians to use acoustical stimulation in reshaping the response of the patients to their tinnitus. The acoustical stimulations can be generated from personal music players, smart phones, and wearable hearing devices and sound generators (Figure 7.3). Most of the advanced sound generators can be digitally programmed by audiologists based on the data from the

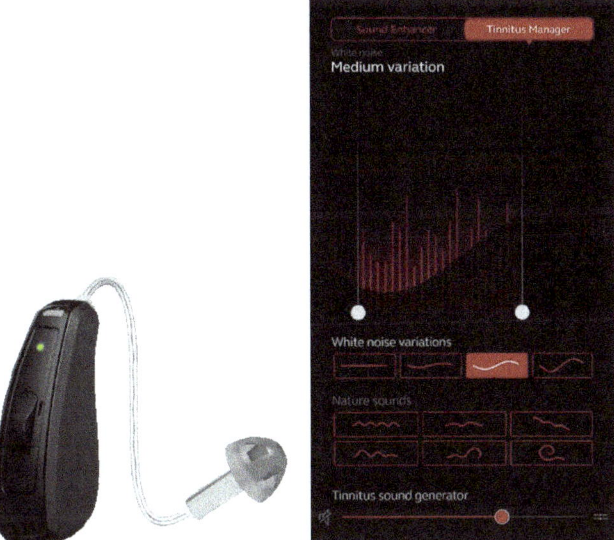

Fig. 7.3 A wearable digital tinnitus sound generator and its companion app (from GN ReSound).

psychoacoustic tinnitus assessments, particularly the information about the pitch and loudness of the patient's tinnitus. Advanced sound generators usually have a companion application where the user, to some extent, can modify acoustical stimulations for their spectral pitch, waveform modulations, and loudness. Additionally, for patients with hearing loss and tinnitus, the process of hearing-amplified environmental sounds and speech, via hearing aids, is extremely effective in reducing awareness of tinnitus. Individuals with hearing loss and tinnitus often say that they do not 'hear' their tinnitus particularly if they have used their hearing aids for years. It appears that the compensation for hearing loss provided by the use of hearing aids results in further neuroplasticity of the auditory centers in the brain and when the hearing loss is effectively compensated for, the brain does not look for a phantom sound that we call tinnitus! A tinnitus sound therapy program when combined with counselling and relaxation techniques is a very effective and non-invasive approach in the management of tinnitus. Techniques such as Tinnitus Retraining Therapy,[16] Tinnitus Activities Treatment,[17] and Progressive Tinnitus Management[18] use similar techniques in enhancing coping strategies and habituation to tinnitus.

Cognitive Behavioral Therapy

According to the practice guidelines by the work of Tunkel *et al.*[13] CBT is one of the highest evidence-based approach in the management of tinnitus. The CBT is a psychological technique that emphasizes the relationships between our thoughts, feelings, and behaviors and has been used in the management of many conditions such as pain, anxiety, insomnia, stress, OCD, and tinnitus. Simply put, what we think influences what we do and what we feel. A tinnitus CBT program is made of multiple sessions and it is usually performed by a psychologist; however, there are very few psychologists who have knowledge about tinnitus and there has been a need for audiologists to implement CBT for tinnitus. An audiologist-delivered CBT for tinnitus is a process where patients with tinnitus are trained to identify their negative thoughts about tinnitus, evaluate them, and respond to it. Patients are trained to design a behavioral experiment and to identify if their negative thoughts are justified. Here are two examples of the negative thoughts that clinicians may hear from their patients: 'my family will be better off without me' or 'I am petrified that tinnitus is going to take over my life.' Hearing such comments from tinnitus patients completely makes sense why the CBT is based on the concepts of thoughts, behaviors, and emotions. A negative thought generates an emotional reaction, which in turn results in behaviors such as avoidance and fear, commonly seen in tinnitus patients. Aazh *et al.*[19] offered the formulation of such negative thoughts resulting in tinnitus-induced distress (Figure 7.4).

In addition to in-person CBT, advances have been made in offering Internet-based CBT (iCBT) for tinnitus. The iCBT for tinnitus can be unguided, where the patient will complete a series of modules for tinnitus management alone or the iCBT can be guided with the assistance from a psychologist or an audiologist trained in CBT. Self-help guides for CBT for tinnitus can also be helpful for some patients.[20]

A patient-friendly and simple model of tinnitus management which addresses the three dimensions of sensation, emotion, and cognition has been proposed and used by the authors (Figure 7.5). In this approach the three factors of sensation, emotion, and cognition are addressed and

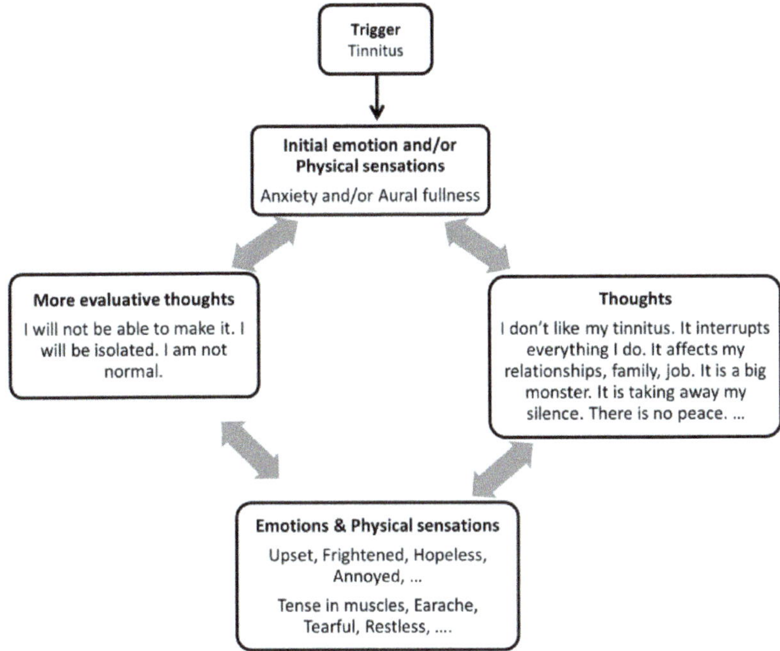

Fig. 7.4 Formulation of distress caused by tinnitus where it is triggered by negative thoughts, triggering emotional reactions, and consequent behaviors.

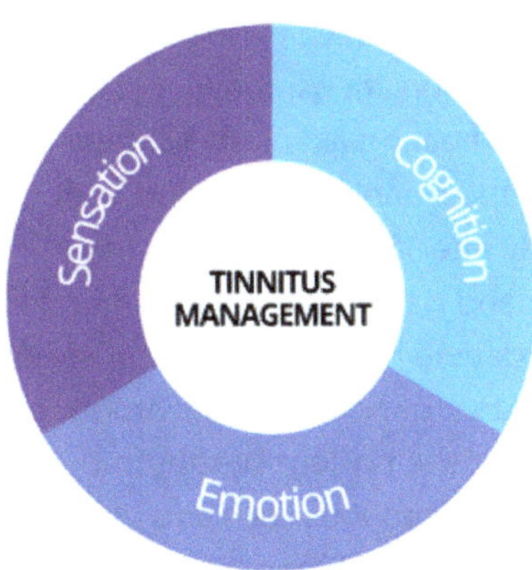

Fig. 7.5 A tinnitus management model that addresses the sensation, emotion, and cognition aspects of tinnitus.

explained to the patients to help them comprehend and absorb how their tinnitus management can be accomplished through the three components of this management plan.

Principles of this approach are developed based on the information that is collected from the patient during their initial interview; completion of tinnitus-related questionnaires; and the data from audiologic and tinnitus assessments. Following assuring the patient that his or her tinnitus is not a life-threatening condition and explaining that all of the potential underlying medical factors have been cleared by their physicians, the patient's tinnitus management is tailored based on their needs in multiple face-to-face sessions and with the use of proper acoustic stimulations.

Sensation

Many patients with tinnitus are annoyed by the sound of it. They describe it as a piercing sound that they perceive deep in their ears or head. Depending on the patient's hearing loss, they are fit with hearing devices that either have amplification only, a sound generator only, or a combination of both amplification and sound generator. Advanced hearing devices give clinicians the flexibility to apply modifications to the sounds and digitally manipulate them according to the patient's needs. Those with hearing loss are instructed to use hearing devices for a few hours a day at the beginning and then increase the use of the devices for the whole day or awake hours. It is explained to the patient with both hearing loss and tinnitus that if they struggle to hear daily conversations, the first sound they will notice is their own tinnitus. This is why hearing aids work for tinnitus patients with hearing loss because they let their tinnitus be mixed with the amplified environmental sounds. Usually after a few months patients in this category do not perceive their tinnitus and gain control over it. For patients with essentially normal hearing or borderline hearing loss, a sound generator is a beneficial tool to use. These sound generators can produce acoustic signals that are spectrally shaped for the patient based on the patient's tinnitus pitch match, or they can generate sounds such as a variety of spectral noise (e.g., white noise, pink or brown noise), frequency-modulated ocean sounds, or fractal music. Many patients report that listening to these sounds soothes their tinnitus and takes the edge off it! Patients use the sound generator devices a few hours a day at the beginning and increase its use to more hours or just use them in quiet places or when they sleep. It usually takes a year for patients to habituate to their tinnitus and they may not need to use the sound generators anymore or use it as needed.

Emotion

Emotional reactions to tinnitus are very common. Patients report sadness, tension, stress, poor sleep habits, fatigue, and feeling down, just to name a few. Being a good listener from the clinician's side and using counselling and relaxation techniques are very important. The impact of tinnitus on daily activities can be enormous and empathy and compassionate care in addition to the application of suitable clinical skills are extremely helpful. It is important for the patient to understand why they show emotional reactions and how to control them. The role of the autonomic nervous system and its subsystems, which include sympathetic and parasympathetic neural pathways, need to be explained to the patient. Patients should be explained about the changes in their emotions when they are under pressure and how the sympathetic nervous system activation can change their patterns of breathing, heartbeat, calmness, or even their voice quality and how the activation of the parasympathetic nervous system can cool down such reactions. When the excitatory and inhibitory roles of these systems are revealed to the patient, they learn how to control them. Application of relaxation techniques including breathing exercises and muscle relaxation is very important. Deep breathing cools down our emotional reaction and reduces our stress level and it is helpful in controlling our reaction to tinnitus and frankly to any other obnoxious signal. There are many apps that can be used to train overly reactive patients how to do proper deep breathing, which is essential for calming them down (Figure 7.6).

In addition to emotional reactions to tinnitus, sleep disturbance can be a major issue for patients with tinnitus. Many complain that tinnitus interferes with their sleep. Good sleeping habits such as avoiding excessive eating before bedtime and listening to soothing sounds while practicing deep breathing can be helpful. Patients need to understand that avoiding excessive noise by protecting their hearing is as important as avoiding quiet places. Damage due to noise can result in changes in the auditory

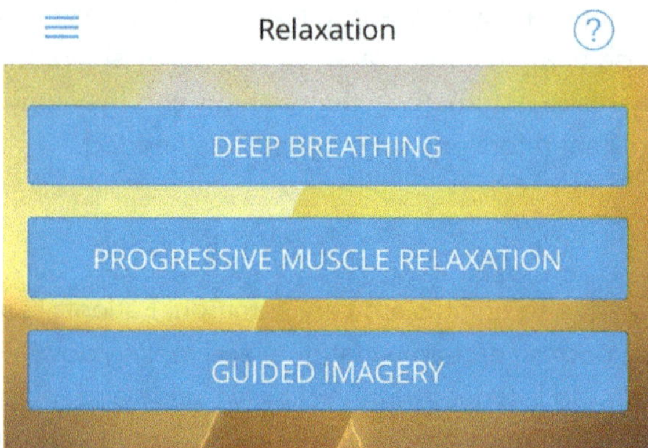

Fig. 7.6 Applications for breathing techniques are useful tools to reduce emotional reactions to tinnitus (from Widex Zen app).

system, which in turn can cause tinnitus. In the same way, patients need to understand that staying in quiet places will make them more aware of their tinnitus. A sound-enriched environment can very effectively distract them from the piercing tinnitus that they experience.

Cognition

This portion of the tinnitus management model discusses the negative thoughts associated with tinnitus. As mentioned in the section for CBT, our thoughts, feelings, and behaviors work together in our perception of tinnitus. Many patients have rumination of negative thoughts. Psychologists define rumination as behaviors associated with repetitive negative thoughts that loops continuously in the mind and never ends. Patients show behaviors such as worrying about an event that may never happen, which in turn can cause mental fatigue and a variety of mental health issues such as anxiety, depression, and stress. Therapeutic exploration of negative thoughts and use of CBT techniques such as behavioral experiments and development of counterstatements for such negative thoughts are formulated for the patients. The CBT for tinnitus is usually offered under the supervision of psychologists familiar with tinnitus or properly CBT-trained audiologists. Adding CBT and iCBT modules combined with sound therapy and emotional reaction control techniques offers a smooth path for recovery for many patients.

Supplements for Tinnitus

The search for a magic pill for tinnitus has been a long journey. It is the nature of humans to find the easiest and fastest way to solve a problem and unfortunately, at least for now, tinnitus is not one of the conditions that can have a *magic pill* or a *quick fix* approach! There is not much evidence that any specific supplement alone works for tinnitus; however, use of antioxidants (vitamins A, C and E and vegetables such as broccoli and sprouts), Japanese garlic (magic medicine), Moringa supplements, zinc and lipoflavonoids can be potentially useful for a better cochlear health and blood circulation. Medical professionals may also use medications that can reduce the comorbid factors associated with tinnitus such as anxiety, tension, stress, depression, and insomnia. Although these medications do not fully address tinnitus, they may contribute to reduction of its consequences or associative factors.

Various supplements may dampen the effects of tinnitus, but some run the risk of side effects. Stress on the cochlea and inner ear structures is thought to play a role in the development of tinnitus.[21] Many proposed treatments thus focus on eliminating the molecular products caused by this stress. In this line of research, authors have recommended usage of various type of antioxidants with mixed outcomes. For example, in a recent study, antioxidant supplementation with acai extract was found to reduce levels of tinnitus.[22] Increasingly growing in popularity, acai is a fruit originating in Brazil with known antioxidant properties.[22] Taking 100 mg capsules of acai extract per day yielded no side effects in study participants.[22] Vitamin B12 deficiency also can increase free radicals that could potentially impact tinnitus. Patients in a study with both B12 deficiency and tinnitus were given B12 injections over a period of 6 weeks.[23] Although these studies show some success, this treatment is for a specific B12-deficient subgroup and would not be applicable to everyone with tinnitus. Melatonin is also potentially helpful, specifically in elderly patients with lower natural levels or individuals who have difficulty falling asleep.[23] As for side effects, there is a report of increased nightmares. However, the effectiveness of melatonin has not been firmly established since studies may be exaggerating its effects on tinnitus.[23] Older patients may also have lower levels of zinc.[23] Zinc supplementation has been considered in the treatment of tinnitus, but the results are mixed. Some studies found no significant association between zinc supplementation and tinnitus outcomes.[24] Even though Zinc is naturally present in the body and serves important purposes, it is a heavy metal that can have toxic effects at 200 mg or more per day, which must be considered in patients looking to supplement with it.[23] While some studies seem promising, zinc as treatment for tinnitus should be studied in more depth because of its potential harmfulness at high dose.

Looking to alternative medicine, Korean red ginseng (KRG), *Ginkgo biloba*, and Gushen Pian each may have significantly positive effects on tinnitus.[23,25] KRG has been found to reduce persistent tinnitus, but only significantly when also administered with *Ginkgo biloba*.[25] KRG may cause side effects such as vomiting, diarrhea, insomnia, mania, vaginal bleeding, breast pain, and blood pressure shift.[26] This is a common concern with regard to many supplements, as they are not as strictly regulated by institutional agencies such as the FDA. *Ginkgo biloba* is a more commonly used supplement in the treatment of tinnitus. It is traditionally used in Chinese medicine and has flavonoids and terpenoids as part of its make-up.[23] However, some Ginkgo supplements may not be purified enough to the correct composition and will thus not have the intended therapeutic impact as it is suggested by many authors.[23]

Acupuncture

Acupuncture is a treatment in traditional Chinese medicine that involves placing needles in predetermined acupuncture points on the body.[27] While some success is noted in the literature coming from Asia, some argue that these studies have inherent flaws as they are not based on evidence-based medicine as it is practiced in the Western world, thus discrediting the results.[23] In some of these studies with positive results, it was found that continued acupuncture is necessary to maintain tinnitus management.[27] Many found that multiple sessions are necessary to see any effect.[23] It was suggested that the positive effect may be related to release of endorphins during the needle acupuncture combined with the relaxation (and anti-stress effect) that results from these sessions. While acupuncture is an interesting treatment to consider, more studies are necessary using the appropriate double-blind clinical trial to measure their effects and ruling out the placebo effect alone, even in light of some positive results.[28] We have noticed in our own practice some positive effect once acupuncture is combined with auriculotherapy mainly for patients suffering from somatosensory tinnitus. The main acupuncture points proposed are the following: Shen Men, LI-4, and KI-3. It is suggested by some authors to use a strong stimulation with a filiform needles or electric acupuncture once daily or every other day. It should also be noted that in case of somatosensory tinnitus, management of an associated TMJ disorders (temporomandibular joint disorder) will have a positive effect on many patients.

Steroid Treatments

Steroid injections also have potential to diminish levels of tinnitus and may be an effective medical therapy in certain patients. The steroid can be administered orally (i.e., prednisone) or more commonly is injected in the middle ear (i.e., dexamethasone), and these intratympanic dexamethasone (ITD) injections have shown some level of efficacy in relieving tinnitus.[29] ITD injections given to patients suffering from tinnitus yielded promising results. In a sample size of 40 patients, 60% showed complete resolution and another 25% showed partial improvement.[29] As with other treatments, there is no guarantee that intratympanic steroid injections will lead to complete resolution of tinnitus. Nevertheless, this therapeutic option should be considered due to its potential to help patients suffering from this prevalent problem, particularly when the tinnitus is of recent onset and related to a sudden hearing loss or noise trauma.

Cochlear Implant Surgery

A more interesting approach to the treatment of tinnitus is cochlear implantation (CI).[30,31] This method is particularly useful in patients dealing with tinnitus when associated with significant hearing loss, with rates of tinnitus improvement anywhere between 68% and 100%.[32,33] The exact mechanism of partial tinnitus evolvement post-implantation is still being studied. A meta-analysis on the association between CI and tinnitus solidified the argument that CI can significantly affect tinnitus outcomes. In six studies, THI scores showed a statistically significant decrease after CI.[32] A 2023 study further solidified the evidence on CI and its mostly positive effects on tinnitus. In this longitudinal study, patients with sensorineural hearing loss had their tinnitus tracked pre- and post-surgery using the Danish THI and the Visual Analogue Scale. Patients with higher initial scores on these scales showed the most tinnitus improvement post-implantation.[33] These studies provide insight into the potential usefulness of CI for the management of tinnitus, particularly in patients who need a cochlear implant for severe to profound hearing loss.

Hyperacusis and Other Decreased Sound Tolerance Disorders

Definition of Hyperacusis

There are many definitions for hyperacusis. In general, clinicians believe that the definition for hyperacusis should include decreased tolerance and oversensitivity to the loudness of sounds which cause distress to the individuals. According to Tyler *et al.*[34] there are four classes of hyperacusis. The first type is *Loudness Hyperacusis,* where the sound tolerance to moderately loud sounds is diminished and uncomfortable. The second type of hyperacusis is referred to as *Annoyance Hyperacusis* and may also be called *Misophonia*. Those who suffer from this condition are not really annoyed by the loudness of the sounds but by their content, meaning, and repetitiveness. Biologic sounds such as chewing, breathing, coughing and throat clearing, and belching along with some non-biologic sounds such as tapping, pen clicking, or computer keyboard sounds are some examples of annoying sounds for those in this category. The third class is *Fear Hyperacusis*, which some may refer to as *Phonophobia*. Those with this class of hyperacusis show avoidance behaviors and try to isolate themselves from any surrounding sounds. The individuals in this category walk around with a pair of headphones or earplugs practically all the time. The fourth class of hyperacusis is referred to as *Pain Hyperacusis*. Those in this category usually have a very decreased tolerance to the sounds where even a normal level of conversational speech or their own voice are considered as painful. One may explain this phenomenon as the auditory signals being sent to the brain as pain signals.

Causes of Hyperacusis and Other Types of Decreased Sound Tolerance Disorders

The etiology of hyperacusis includes a variety of factors and it is not a homogenic disorder; therefore, many causes are attributed to its generation. It seems that the most common cause of hyperacusis is noise exposure. However, factors such as aging, medications, anxiety, migraine, Bell's palsy, head traumas, superior semicircular canal dehiscence, and TMJ involvement are some other causes of hyperacusis. For many patients, hyperacusis is associated with tinnitus. Those with both tinnitus and hyperacusis may report more annoyance from one or the other condition.

Assessment and Intervention for Hyperacusis and Other Types of Decreased Sound Tolerance Disorders

Hyperacusis assessment starts with a comprehensive case history in order to pinpoint underlying pathologies that may contribute to this. Use of questionnaires such as Hyperacusis Questionnaire[35] and Inventory of Hyperacusis Symptoms[36] can help in the assessment of the impact on the quality of life of those who suffer from hyperacusis. A comprehensive audiologic examination including the measurement of loudness discomfort levels across a variety of frequencies is very essential. Figure 7.7 shows the audiometric

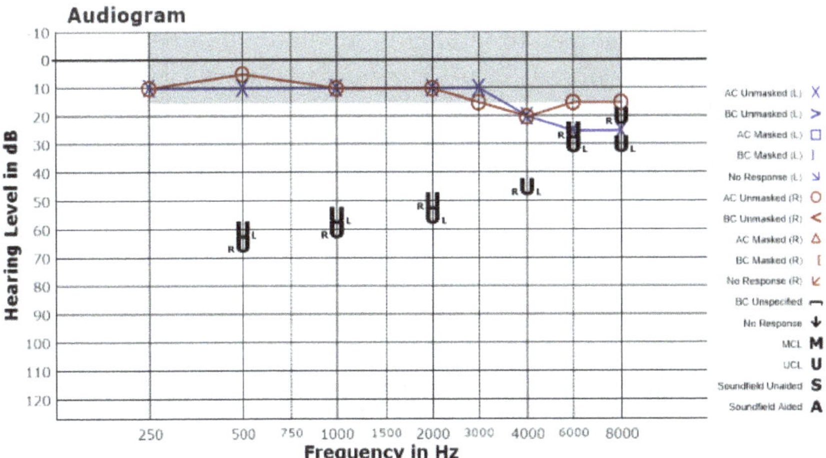

Fig. 7.7 Hyperacusis audiogram representing a severe case.

data of a patient with severe hyperacusis following a head trauma after a car accident. As can be seen, the patient has a very diminished tolerance to the sounds, particularly at higher frequencies.

Intervention for Hyperacusis and Misophonia

Management of decreased sound tolerance disorders is essentially very similar to the management of tinnitus. Techniques of CBT, sound therapy, and counselling have been used to help in the intervention process of hyperacusis and misophonia.[37] For hyperacusis, gradual increments in the acoustical signals delivered via the sound generators can increase the patient's tolerance to the sounds in a majority of cases. The practical model of tinnitus management that addresses sensation, emotion, and cognition (Figure 7.5) can be adopted in helping patients who suffer from hyperacusis and misophonia as well. Patients are advised that sensitivity to external sounds (i.e., hyperacusis and misophonia) is very similar to sensitivity to internally generated sounds (i.e., tinnitus); therefore, the management strategies essentially use similar protocols.

References

1. Dietrich S. (2004) Earliest historic reference of 'tinnitus' is controversial. *J Laryngol Otol* **118**(7):487–8.
2. Azizi MH. (2007) The otorhinolaryngologic concepts as viewed by Rhazes and Avicenna. *Arch Iran Med* **10**(4):552–5.
3. Erlandsson S, Dauman N. (2013) Categorization of tinnitus in view of history and medical discourse. *Int J Qual Stud Health Well-being* **8**:23530.
4. InformedHealth.org. (2006) *Tinnitus: Overview* [Internet]. Cologne, Germany: Institute for Quality and Efficiency in Health Care (IQWiG). 2008 Aug 25 [Updated 2019 Mar 28]. Available at: https://www.ncbi.nlm.nih.gov/books/NBK395560/
5. Wells HRR, Abidin FNZ, Freidin MB, *et al.* (2021) Genome-wide association study suggests that variation at the RCOR1 locus is associated with tinnitus in UK Biobank. *Sci Rep* **11**(1):6470. doi:10.1038/s41598-021-85871-6
6. Soni A, Dubey A. (2020) Chronic primary tinnitus: A management dilemma. *Audiol Res* **10**(2):55–66.

7. Henry JA, Roberts LE, Caspary DM, *et al.* (2014) Underlying mechanisms of tinnitus: Review and clinical implications. *J Am Acad Audiol* **25**(1):5–22.
8. Newman CW, Jacobson GP, Spitzer JB. (1996) Development of the tinnitus handicap inventory. *Arch Otolaryngol Head Neck Surg* **122**(2):143–8.
9. Meikle MB, Henry JA, Griest SE, *et al.* (2012) The tinnitus functional index: Development of a new clinical measure for chronic, intrusive tinnitus. *Ear Hear* **33**(2):153–76.
10. Aazh H, Hayes C, Moore BCJ, Vitoratou S. (2022) Psychometric evaluation of the tinnitus impact questionnaire using patients seeking help for tinnitus or tinnitus with hyperacusis. *Int J Audiol* 1–10. doi:10.1080/14992027.2022.2101027. Epub ahead of print. PMID: 35916560.
11. Lockwood AH, Wack DS, Burkard RF, *et al.* (2001) The functional anatomy of gaze-evoked tinnitus and sustained lateral gaze. *Neurology* **56**(4):472–80.
12. Danesh A, Kinouchi Y, Wener D, Pandya A. (2003) Functional imaging of tinnitus: seeing of the unseeable. In: Palade V, Howlett RJ, Jain LC (eds.), *Proceedings of KES 2003 Seventh International Conference on Knowledge-Based Intelligent Information and Engineering Systems*. Berlin: Springer-Verlag, pp. 794–799.
13. Tunkel DE, Bauer CA, Sun GH, *et al.* (2014) Clinical practice guideline: Tinnitus. *Otolaryngol Head Neck Surg* **151**(2 Suppl):S1–40. doi:10.1177/0194599814545325. PMID: 25273878.
14. Denton AJ, Finberg A, Ashman PE, *et al.* (2021) Implications of transcranial magnetic stimulation as a treatment modality for tinnitus. *J Clin Med* **10**(22):5422. doi:10.3390/jcm10225422. PMID: 34830704; PMCID: PMC8622674.
15. Conlon B, Langguth B, Hamilton C, *et al.* (2020) Bimodal neuromodulation combining sound and tongue stimulation reduces tinnitus symptoms in a large randomized clinical study. *Sci Transl Med* **12**(564):eabb2830. doi:10.1126/scitranslmed.abb2830. PMID: 33028707.
16. Jastreboff PJ, Jastreboff MM. (2006) Tinnitus retraining therapy: a different view on tinnitus. *ORL J Otorhinolaryngol Relat Spec* **68**(1):23–9; discussion 29–30. doi:10.1159/000090487. Epub 2006 Mar 3. PMID: 16514259.
17. Tyler RS, Gogel SA, Gehringer AK. (2007) Tinnitus activities treatment. *Prog Brain Res* **166**:425–34. doi:10.1016/S0079-6123(07)66041-5. PMID: 17956807.
18. Henry JA, Zaugg TL, Myers PJ, Schechter MA. (2008) The role of audiologic evaluation in progressive audiologic tinnitus management. *Trends Amplif*

12(3):170–87. doi:10.1177/1084713808319941. Epub 2008 Jul 15. PMID: 18628281; PMCID: PMC4134888.

19. Aazh H, Landgrebe M, Danesh AA, Moore BC. (2019) Cognitive behavioral therapy for alleviating the distress caused by tinnitus, hyperacusis and misophonia: Current perspectives. *Psychol Res Behav Manag* **12**:991–1002. doi:10.2147/PRBM.S179138. PMID: 31749641; PMCID: PMC6817772.
20. Aazh H, Moore BCJ. (2022) *Living Well with Tinnitus: A Self-Help Guide Using Cognitive Behavioural Therapy.* London, UK: Little, Brown Book Group.
21. Petridou AI, Zagora ET, Petridis P, *et al.* (2019) The effect of antioxidant supplementation in patients with tinnitus and normal hearing or hearing loss: a randomized, double-blind, placebo controlled trial. *Nutrients* **11**(12):3037. doi:10.3390/nu11123037. PMID: 31842394; PMCID: PMC6950042.
22. Oppitz SJ, Garcia MV, Bruno RS, *et al.* (2022) Supplementation with açaí (Euterpe Oleracea Martius) for the treatment of chronic tinnitus: Effects on perception, anxiety levels and oxidative metabolism biomarkers. *CoDAS* **34**(4):e20210076. doi:10.1590/2317-1782/20212021076. PMID: 35107519; PMCID: PMC9886123.
23. Luetzenberg FS, Babu S, Seidman MD. (2020) Alternative treatments of tinnitus: Alternative medicine. *Otolaryngol Clin North Am* **53**(4):637–50. doi:10.1016/j.otc.2020.03.011. Epub 2020 Apr 30. PMID: 32362562.
24. Person OC, Puga MES, da Silva EMK, Torloni MR. (2016) Zinc supplementation for tinnitus. *Cochrane Database Syst Rev* **11**(11):CD009832. doi:10.1002/14651858.CD009832.pub2. Accessed 10 May 2023.
25. Kim TS, Lee HS, Chung JW. (2015) The effect of Korean red ginseng on symptoms and quality of life in chronic tinnitus: A randomized, open-label pilot study. *J Audiol Otol* **19**(2):85–90. doi:10.7874/jao.2015.19.2.85. Epub 2015 Sep 16. PMID: 26413574; PMCID: PMC4582451.
26. Liu L. (2019) Side effects of ginseng supplements. Side Effects of Ginseng. https://www.poison.org/articles/side-effects-of-ginseng-supplements-191
27. Kuzucu I, Karaca O. (2020) Acupuncture treatment in patients with chronic subjective tinnitus: A prospective, randomized study. *Med Acupunct* **32**(1): 24–8. doi:10.1089/acu.2019.1367. Epub 2020 Feb 3. PMID: 32104524; PMCID: PMC7041314.
28. Wu Q, Wang J, Han D, *et al.* (2023) Efficacy and safety of acupuncture and moxibustion for primary tinnitus: A systematic review and meta-analysis. *Am J Otolaryngol* **44**(3):103821. doi:10.1016/j.amjoto.2023.103821. Epub 2023 Feb 26. PMID: 36905913.

29. Sayoo C, Kumar S. (2019) Intratympanic injection of steroid for treatment of tinnitus. *Indian J Otolaryngol Head Neck Surg* **71**(Suppl 2):1123–5. doi:10.1007/s12070-017-1213-3. Epub 2017 Sep 30. PMID: 31750136; PMCID: PMC6841828.
30. Eshraghi AA, Nazarian R, Telischi FF, *et al.* (2012) The cochlear implant: Historical aspects and future prospects. *Anat Rec (Hoboken)* **295**(11):1967–80. doi:10.1002/ar.22580. Epub 2012 Oct 8. PMID: 23044644; PMCID: PMC4921065.
31. Eshraghi AA, Gupta C, Ozdamar O, *et al.* (2012) Biomedical engineering principles of modern cochlear implants and recent surgical innovations. *Anat Rec (Hoboken)* **295**(11):1957–66. doi:10.1002/ar.22584. Epub 2012 Oct 8. PMID: 23044779.
32. Borges ALF, Duarte PLES, Almeida RBS, *et al.* (2021) Cochlear implant and tinnitus-a meta-analysis. *Braz J Otorhinolaryngol* **87**(3):353–65. doi:10.1016/j.bjorl.2020.11.006. Epub 2020 Dec 8. PMID: 33342697; PMCID: PMC9422519.
33. Rasmussen KD, West NC, Bille M, Cayé-Thomasen P. (2023) Tinnitus suppression in a prospective cohort of 45 cochlear implant recipients: occurrence, degree and correlates. *Eur Arch Otorhinolaryngol.* doi:10.1007/s00405-023-07921-1. Epub ahead of print. PMID: 37099145.
34. Tyler RS, Pienkowski M, Roncancio ER, *et al.* (2014) A review of hyperacusis and future directions: part I. Definitions and manifestations. *Am J Audiol* **23**(4):402–19. doi:10.1044/2014_AJA-14-0010. PMID: 25104073.
35. Khalfa S, Dubal S, Veuillet E, *et al.* (2002) Psychometric normalization of a hyperacusis questionnaire. *ORL J Otorhinolaryngol Relat Spec* **64**(6):436–42. doi:10.1159/000067570. PMID: 12499770.
36. Greenberg B, Carlos M. (2018) Psychometric properties and factor structure of a new scale to measure hyperacusis: Introducing the inventory of hyperacusis symptoms. *Ear Hear* **39**(5):1025–34. doi:10.1097/AUD.0000000000000583. PMID: 29742543.
37. Danesh AA, Aazh H. (2020) Misophonia: A neurologic, psychologic, and audiologic complex. *Hear J* **73**:20–3.

8 Novel Immunologic-Related Approaches to Treating Sensorineural Hearing Loss

Ilana Yellin, MD[1]; Andrea Vambutas, MD[1]

Abstract

Immune-mediated inner ear disease (IMED) represents several disease processes, all of which can be characterized by a new, asymmetric sensorineural hearing loss that may be ameliorated by timely immunosuppression. However, not all patients are responsive to corticosteroids. As a result, there is a clear clinical need to identify the mechanisms by which the hearing loss occurs, thereby identifying new potential therapeutic targets for intervention. Furthermore, within IMED, although sudden sensorineural hearing loss (SSNHL) and Meniere's disease (MD) can be clearly characterized, autoimmune inner ear disease (AIED) is a complex entity that presents challenges for both diagnosis and management. While the pathogenesis of disease remains to be fully delineated, proposed pathological mechanisms include immunological perturbations in both the innate and adaptive immune response, vascular compromise, and disturbances in cochlear physiology. First-line treatment for all patients with suspected IMED includes high-dose oral corticosteroids and/or intratympanic steroid injections. The injection alone may provide benefit for those who cannot tolerate systemic treatment. For those who fail to respond or become resistant to steroids, biological agents such as anakinra may offer promising results. Finally, patients with IMED with profound hearing loss should be considered for early cochlear implantation for the best long-term results although their hearing may continue to fluctuate even after implantation.

Corresponding Author: Andrea Vambutas MD

[1] Department of Otolaryngology, Donald and Barbara Zucker School of Medicine at Hofstra-Northwell, New Hyde Park, NY, United States.

Diagnosis and Clinical Presentation

Immune-mediated inner ear disease (IMED) is comprised of all sensorineural hearing losses (SNHLs) that may be potentially reversed by timely corticosteroid treatment or other forms of immunosuppression. Clinical, ear-specific forms of IMED include sudden sensorineural hearing loss (SSNHL), Meniere's disease (MD), and autoimmune inner ear disease (AIED). Of these diseases, AIED is a rare entity that poses a diagnostic challenge. It accounts for <1% of all SNHL and the diagnosis is further complicated by the lack of specific diagnostic tests that rule in disease.[1] The definition of AIED has varied over the last several decades; while response to corticosteroids was previously a requisite for diagnosis, we now understand that a subset of patients with AIED do not symptomatically improve following courses of high-dose steroids, and the majority of AIED patients lose the ability to respond to corticosteroids over time.[2] Manifestations of AIED may be organ specific or associated with systemic autoimmune disease.[3] To complicate matters further, autoinflammatory diseases are systemic diseases of the innate immune system that can involve the auditory system and cause SNHL.[4] These disorders pose similar diagnostic challenges as the clinical presentation and the severity of symptoms is highly variable although genetic testing can provide definitive diagnosis.

A yet-to-be classified orphan disease, AIED has an estimated prevalence of only 15/100,000, or approximately 45,000 persons in the United States at any given time.[4] AIED in conjunction with systemic disease is more frequent than organ-specific AIED and 25–30% of patients with organ-specific AIED will eventually develop symptoms of systemic autoimmune or autoinflammatory disorders as hearing loss may be the first manifestation of systemic disease.[1] In a small series of patients with AIED, Broughton *et al.* found that the onset of vestibuloauditory symptoms preceded the diagnosis of systemic disease in 57% of patients with AIED.[4] Systemic disorders associated with immune-related hearing loss include systemic sclerosis (SS), rheumatoid arthritis (RA), Sjogren's disease, systemic lupus erythematosus (SLE), relapsing polychondritis, Cogan's disease, granulomatosis with polyangiitis, mixed cryoglobulinemia, ulcerative colitis, giant cell arteritis, Behcet's disease, and Vogt–Koyanagi–Harada syndrome. The prevalence of hearing loss varies among these diseases, ranging from 2%

in ulcerative colitis, 21–41% in Cogan's disease, to potentially greater than 50% in SLE and granulomatosis with polyangiitis.[1]

Despite advances in research, there continues to be a lack of consensus for the diagnostic criteria for AIED. The most widely accepted criteria include progressive, bilateral, and asymmetric SNHL of at least 30 dB in one or more frequencies developing over greater than three but less than 90 days.[5] All patients should undergo magnetic resonance imaging (MRI) to rule out retrocochlear pathology. Presentation varies and may be characterized by bilateral sequential or sudden unilateral hearing loss which is typically rapidly progressive and fluctuating.[1] While Malik *et al.* report disease beginning bilaterally in only 23.1%, Broughton *et al.* report 79% of their cohort ultimately suffering from bilateral disease. The median age of hearing loss onset is 50–55 years and both genders are affected equally. Tinnitus and vestibular symptoms are present in 42–83% and 79% of patients, respectively, while 50% of patients fit criteria for MD.[2,3]

Pathogenesis and Molecular Targets

The pathogenesis of AIED has yet to be fully elucidated, and may represent a spectrum of diseases. The disease exhibits features of both autoinflammatory and autoimmune diseases, where autoinflammatory diseases are mediated by monocytes and characterized by low-titer autoantibodies and interleukin-1(IL-1B) release, while autoimmune diseases are mediated by T cells and characterized by high-titer autoantibodies and release of interleukin-17, interferon, and tumor necrosis factor (TNF).[4] Given the wide variety of diseases associated with AIED, various mechanisms of injury have been postulated to result in SNHL. Proposed pathological mechanisms include cytokine dysregulation, self-reactive T cells and immunoglobulins, immune-complex deposition, microthrombosis, and electrochemical disturbances in the cochlea causing impaired neurosignalling.[6]

Given the limited access to the human cochlea, much of our understanding relating to the pathogenesis of AIED comes from animal models inoculated with keyhole limpet hemocyanin (KLH), an immunogen used to induce labyrinthitis. These animal models demonstrate an upregulation of TNF and IL-1B, which in turn causes T-cell switching to a Th-1 response and perpetuates an autoimmune response through release of interferon gamma.[6] The upregulation of IL-1B plays a key role in Muckle–Wells disease, an autoinflammatory disorder caused by a gain of function mutation in NLRP-3 resulting in SNHL and systemic amyloidosis. Understanding the role of IL-1B in the pathogenesis of AIED has important implications for identifying molecular targets for treatment as patients with SNHL associated with Muckle–Wells disease experience improved or stabilized hearing with IL-1B inhibition by anakinra.[4]

Additional animal models have also implicated antibody formation and circulating immune complexes in the pathogenesis of AIED. In murine models with lymphoproliferative disorders and prone to autoimmune diseases, hearing loss was associated with degeneration of the stria vascularis secondary to immune complex deposition.[6] This damage to the stria vascularis is consistent with histopathological changes seen in patients with polyarteritis nodosa, and ultimately results in changes to electrochemical gradients in the cochlea, which in turn disrupts nerve signaling.[1,6] Immune complex deposition affecting the microvascular environment of the cochlea is again implicated in the pathogenesis of SNHL in patients with RA, Hashimoto's disease, and mixed cryoglobulinemia. In antiphospholipid syndrome, antibodies are thought to result in microthromboses affecting the cochlea and may be successfully treated with enoxaparin.[1,6]

Numerous vestibulocochlear antigens and autoantibodies have been identified among AIED patients but there has yet to be a single autoantibody identified among all patients. Among those first identified is HSP70, an autoantibody against a 68 kDa that was initially thought to predict steroid responsiveness. It is found in only 35% of AIED patients and has subsequently been detected in control patients at a similar rate. Furthermore, it is not specific to the inner ear and is also found in the brain and muscle.[6] Other identified antibodies include anti-myelin P0 antibodies, which have been validated as a marker of vestibular failure, and anti-B actin antibodies, which have been correlated with audiovestibular dysfunction in animals. Finally, antibodies specific to the inner ear which have been identified in animal models include anti-cochlin, anti-KHRI-3, and anti-connexin-26 antibodies.[6]

Clinical Management

Steroids

Immune-mediated inner ear disease is the only form of SNHL that is responsive to medical therapy and oral corticosteroids remain first-line treatment for SSNHL and AIED. While response to corticosteroids had historically been a requisite for diagnosis of AIED, response rates are variable and upon initial treatment may be as high as 70%.[4] The standard treatment is typically 1 mg/kg/day of prednisone with an upper limit of 60 mg/day. Responders are identified as those with a threshold shift of ≥15 dB at one frequency, ≥10 dB across two or more consecutive frequencies, or a 12% increase in word recognition score (WRS).[5]

The mechanism by which corticosteroid treatment results in clinical improvement in some patients is not yet fully elucidated. Animal studies suggest that corticosteroids act by binding mineralocorticoid receptors to restore imbalances in electrochemical gradients in the cochlea while human studies have demonstrated normalization of T-cell expression in steroid responders.[6] There is also evidence to suggest that steroids act by modulating IL-1B expression. In a small subset of patients with end-stage AIED undergoing cochlear implant, steroid treatment was associated with increased expression of IL-1R2, a decoy receptor that sequesters IL-1B preventing downstream signaling and inflammation. Additionally, steroid responders had low basal levels of IL-1R2, which dramatically increased with steroid treatment while steroid non-responders had high basal levels of IL-1R2, which minimally changed with steroid treatment. These observations suggest that endogenous IL-1B was expressed in those patients who failed to respond to corticosteroids with concomitant IL-1R2 expression, and that corticosteroids induced decoy receptor expression which specifically correlated with clinical hearing improvement.[7]

While steroids initially offer promising results to 50–70% of patients, only 14% remain responsive after 34 months.[2] Furthermore, the long-term use of oral steroids is problematic due to their associated systemic side effects. For this reason, intratympanic corticosteroid injection may be a suitable alternative for those who cannot tolerate systemic treatment. Intratympanic injections allow for increased concentrations of drug to reach the perilymph without the risk of systemic side effects. Intratympanic steroids have been shown to be as effective as oral steroids for the management of idiopathic SNHL, but it remains unclear if there are any distinct advantages for their use in the treatment of AIED.[4] Adjunct use of N-acetylcysteine (NAC) with corticosteroids has been demonstrated to be beneficial in SSNHL improved hearing recovery, as well as in hearing preservation post-cochlear implantation.[8] In peripheral blood immune cells from AIED patients, NAC reduces TNF in corticosteroid-responsive patients.

Biologics and Non-Steroidal Alternatives

There are no universal guidelines for the management of AIED in patients who cannot maintain their response with the discontinuation of corticosteroids, do not respond to corticosteroids, or become resistant to corticosteroids. Alternative treatments including methotrexate, cyclophosphamide, TNF-α inhibitors, and IL-1B antagonists have been trialed with varying success.[4,5,9,10]

Historically, cyclophosphamide, an alkylating agent inhibiting protein synthesis, had been used in conjunction with steroids and was associated with improvement in pure tone average (PTA) and WRS. However, the drug is no longer used in the treatment of AIED given its poor side effect profile.[2] Methotrexate has a better side effect profile and has been reported to improve vestibular symptoms in 80–100% of patients but is not effective in maintaining long-term hearing outcomes.[2,5]

In a phase I/II open label, single-arm clinical trial, anakinra demonstrated clinical efficacy in a small sample of steroid-resistant patients.[9] Anakinra is an IL-1B receptor antagonist that inhibits IL-1B binding to its cognate receptor. The patients were given daily subcutaneous injections of 100 mg of anakinra for 84 days and followed for an additional 180 days. In patients who responded to anakinra, there was a reduction in plasma IL-1β, which correlated with clinical improvement. Furthermore, relapse in symptoms was associated with a rise in IL-1β plasma levels.[9] Interestingly, in Muckle–Wells disease, an autoinflammatory disease caused by a gain-of function mutation that results in excessive IL-1B, use of anakinra largely resulted in maintenance of hearing rather than clinical improvement although case reports of hearing improvement have been published.[4]

Alternative biological agents such as those in the class of TNF-α inhibitors have shown varying efficacy. In a guinea pig model inoculated with KLH to induce labyrinthitis, TNF was robustly expressed in cochlear immunocytes and suppressed with etanercept; however, the results did not translate into a meaningful hearing improvement for patients with AIED. In an open-label pilot study where 23 patients were treated with biweekly 25 mg subcutaneous injections of etanercept, only 30% of patients had improvement in hearing.[10] However, caution should be exercised in discarding anti-TNF therapies from treating AIED. There have been two trials investigating intratympanic use of TNF-α inhibitors including golimumab and infliximab, both of which allowed for full steroid tapering without loss of hearing function in almost all steroid-dependent AIED patients studied. TNF inhibition has also been demonstrated to be beneficial in Cogan's disease, a rare autoimmune disease with cochlea-vestibular dysfunction and ocular disease.

While each of these studies focuses on a small subset of patients, larger studies are difficult, given the extreme rarity of the disease. As patients become resistant to oral corticosteroids, unable to maintain hearing with the discontinuation of corticosteroids, or unable to tolerate the complications with ongoing corticosteroid use, the clinical need to identify biological targets for potential alternatives is crucial. Unfortunately, our ability to do so is hindered by our limited access to the human cochlea. Many of the molecular targets identified in animal models of cochlear inflammation have not translated into improved therapies for human disease. Although the cochlea was believed to be immunologically privileged and impervious to the peripheral immune system, we now know that peripheral immune cells access many of these privileged sites such as the brain, the eye, and the cochlea. As such, studies of the peripheral blood immune cells of AIED patients have elucidated molecular targets, as has perilymph sampling from the cochlea of these patients undergoing cochlear implantation.[7,9]

Implications for Cochlear Implantation

Many patients with AIED become excellent candidates for cochlear implantation as they develop progressive SNHL after decades of hearing. With only a small percentage of patients continuing to benefit from oral corticosteroids after 34 months and unclear efficacy of many biological agents, cochlear implantation is an important option for many patients with AIED suffering from severe or profound SNHL. Early, unilateral implantation provides a safety net for these patients, as the frequency and timing of contralateral ear progression is highly variable. However, the presence of systemic autoimmune disease does have implications for cochlear implant performance.

In a subset of patients with AIED, Malik *et al.* found that 16% of patients had cochlear scarring on MRI prior to cochlear implantation.[3] Additionally, patients with systemic AIED were found to have bone obliteration of the round window and ossification of the basal turn of the cochlea.[1] Cochlear fibrosis and ossification have been reported to affect up to 50% of AIED-implanted ears and can result in incomplete electrode insertion into the cochlea and less-than-ideal hearing outcomes.[1,3] These findings may explain why better speech perception with cochlear implantation in AIED patients was associated with earlier age at implantation and organ-specific AIED.[3]

Early implantation does not necessarily guarantee long-term results as local relapsing inflammatory responses may induce episodic deterioration or improvement in implant performance. We have observed some AIED patients continue to experience hearing fluctuation post-cochlear implantation, and this should be investigated if the patient experiences a change in their implant performance. Some patients with AIED related to Cogan's syndrome and other systemic autoimmune diseases have documented worsening in post-implant speech recognition scores which may be related to histological manifestations of AIED that continue to progress beyond implantation. These histological changes include degeneration of the spiral ganglion cells, cystic degeneration of the stria vascularis, and vasculitis of the internal auditory canal.[1] In light of the potential for disease progression, early cochlear implantation in this population, before any cochlear destruction or remodeling, is preferred as this increases the likelihood of complete electrode insertion and improved long-term hearing.

Conclusion

Autoimmune inner ear disease is a rare cause of SNHL that can be difficult for the otolaryngologist to both diagnose and treat. Without formal diagnostic criteria, the diagnosis is one of exclusion, recognized by clinical symptoms consisting of progressive, bilateral, and asymmetric SNHL with MRI excluding retrocochlear pathology. The disease may be specific to the inner ear or associated with systemic diseases and while the pathogenesis remains to be fully understood, it exhibits features of both autoinflammatory and autoimmune diseases. Proposed pathological mechanisms include cytokine dysregulation, self-reactive T cells and immunoglobulins, immune-complex deposition, microthrombosis, and electrochemical disturbances in the cochlea causing impaired neurosignaling.

High-dose oral corticosteroids remain the gold standard for treatment and should be initiated in all patients with suspected AIED. Failure to respond to corticosteroids does not rule out AIED, as the majority of patients will eventually become resistant to corticosteroid treatment several years after initial diagnosis if their hearing continues to fluctuate. Intratympanic steroids may be beneficial in those who cannot tolerate systemic treatment. While there are no universal guidelines for the management of AIED in patients who do not respond or become resistant to steroids, various biological agents have been trialed and initial results with anakinra suggested efficacy which is being verified in a larger placebo-controlled trial. Ultimately, some patients with AIED progress to severe-to-profound SNHL and become candidates for cochlear implantation. In this subset of patients, the surgeon should consider early implantation to increase the likelihood of full electrode insertion and improved long-term results.

References

1. Mancini P, Atturo F, Di Mario A, *et al.* (2018) Hearing loss in autoimmune disorders: Prevalence and therapeutic options. *Autoimmun Rev* **17**(7):644–52. doi:10.1016/j.autrev.2018.01.014. Epub 2018 May 3. PMID: 29729446.
2. Broughton SS, Meyerhoff WE, Cohen SB. (2004) Immune-mediated inner ear disease: 10-year experience. *Semin Arthritis Rheum* **34**(2):544–8. doi:10.1016/j.semarthrit.2004.07.001. PMID: 15505770.
3. Malik MU, Pandian V, Masood H, *et al.* (2012) Spectrum of immune-mediated inner ear disease and cochlear implant results. *Laryngoscope* **122**(11):2557–62. doi:10.1002/lary.23604. Epub 2012 Sep 18. PMID: 22991211.

4. Vambutas A, Pathak S. (2016) AAO: Autoimmune and autoinflammatory (disease) in otology: What is new in immune-mediated hearing loss. *Laryngoscope Investig Otolaryngol* **1**(5):110–5. doi:10.1002/lio2.28. Epub 2016 Sep 21. PMID: 27917401; PMCID: PMC5113311.
5. Harris JP, Weisman MH, Derebery JM, *et al.* (2003) Treatment of corticosteroid-responsive autoimmune inner ear disease with methotrexate: A randomized controlled trial. *JAMA* **290**(14):1875–83. doi:10.1001/jama.290.14.1875. Epub 2003 Oct 9; PMID: 14532316.
6. Goodall AF, Siddiq MA. (2015) Current understanding of the pathogenesis of autoimmune inner ear disease: A review. *Clin Otolaryngol* **40**(5):412–9. doi:10.1111/coa.12432. PMID: 25847404.
7. Vambutas A, DeVoti J, Goldofsky E, *et al.* (2009) Alternate splicing of interleukin-1 receptor type II (IL1R2) *in vitro* correlates with clinical glucocorticoid responsiveness in patients with AIED. *PLoS One* **4**(4):e5293. doi:10.1371/journal.pone.0005293. Epub 2009 Apr 29. PMID: 19401759; PMCID: PMC2670509.
8. Eshraghi AA, Roell J, Shaikh N, *et al.* (2016) A novel combination of drug therapy to protect residual hearing post cochlear implant surgery. *Acta Otolaryngol* **136**(4):420–4. doi:10.3109/00016489.2015.1134809. Epub 2016 Feb 9. PMID: 26854005.
9. Vambutas A, Lesser M, Mullooly V, *et al.* (2014) Early efficacy trial of anakinra in corticosteroid-resistant autoimmune inner ear disease. *J Clin Invest* **124**(9):4115–22. doi:10.1172/JCI76503. Epub 2014 Aug 18. PMID: 25133431; PMCID: PMC4160092.
10. Matteson EL, Choi HK, Poe DS, *et al.* (2005) Etanercept therapy for immune-mediated cochleovestibular disorders: A multi-center, open-label, pilot study. *Arthritis Rheum* **53**(3):337–42. doi:10.1002/art.21179. PMID: 15934127.

9 Hearing Aids and Implantable Bone Conduction Devices

Vivian F. Kaul, MD[1]; Bryce P. G. Dzubara, BS[2];
Oliver F. Adunka, MD, MBA[1]

Abstract

Aural rehabilitation can improve quality of life for people of all ages. Devices including hearing aids, implantable hearing aids, bone-anchored hearing aids, cochlear implants, and auditory brainstem implants are some technological advancements in the otologist's/neurotologist's toolbox. Each device has its own set of advantages and limitations, indications and contraindications. Ultimately, the correct device choice for the patient comes down to a team decision, comprised of, but not limited to, the patient, family, audiologist, speech language pathologist, and otologist/neurotologist.

Introduction

Medical devices comprise a diverse array of treatment methods for all forms of hearing loss. Given the many etiologies, mechanisms, and progressions of hearing loss, a period of observation can be a useful component of any treatment plan, and treatment options such as observation, cerumen removal, or pharmacological therapy may be appropriate. Moreover, aural rehabilitation can improve quality of life for patients with hearing loss. However, technological advancements have enabled physicians to treat hearing loss at various points along the auditory pathway in a plethora

---

Corresponding Author: Oliver F. Adunka MD, MBA

[1] Division of Otology, Neurotology and Cranial Base Surgery, Department of Otolaryngology — Head and Neck Surgery, The Ohio State University Wexner Medical Center, Columbus, OH, United States.

[2] Medical School, The Ohio State University, Columbus, OH, United States.

of ways with medical devices. The wide range of treatments provides physicians more options to discuss with patients, ultimately allowing for more appropriate care. This chapter will discuss a few of the major medical device classes currently available, explaining how they work, indications and contraindications for use, and their outcomes in patients.

Hearing Aids

Often the first choice for individuals diagnosed with hearing loss, hearing aids are devices that amplify existing sound. The specific components of hearing aids vary, but most hearing aids are comprised of a small microphone, a battery, an amplifier, and a receiver. The microphone collects sound waves and transmits them to the amplifier, which increases their volume and sends them into the ear to eventually stimulate the cochlear nerve in the cochlea allowing the user to hear the sound.[1] Hearing aids are indicated in almost all patients suffering from sensorineural, mixed, or conductive hearing loss, and different hearing aids are indicated for different ranges of hearing loss.[2] They can also alleviate a patient's tinnitus burden. Typically, a hearing aid trial is undertaken as initial therapy or adjunct concurrent therapy for chronic or progressive hearing loss before moving on to more invasive and expensive options. If a surgical treatment is indicated, and the patient undergoes the procedure, hearing aids may still be utilized after surgery. Hearing aids are contraindicated in patients with chronic middle or outer ear infections and in patients with atresia of the ear canal or other anatomic abnormalities that preclude the fitting and use of conventional hearing aids. Moreover, while not absolutely contraindicated, hearing aids may not benefit patients with severe-to-profound hearing loss due to a low signal-to-noise ratio. As the hearing aids will amplify all environmental sound, patients that require strong amplification will struggle to hear clearly because of the excess background noise that is concurrently being amplified.

With the advancement of hearing aid technology, more individualized treatments are available, and several different types of hearing aids are available today (Figure 9.1). After placement, audiologists can work with patients, adjusting various settings and parameters on the hearing aids to provide the patient with hearing aid performance best suited to their hearing

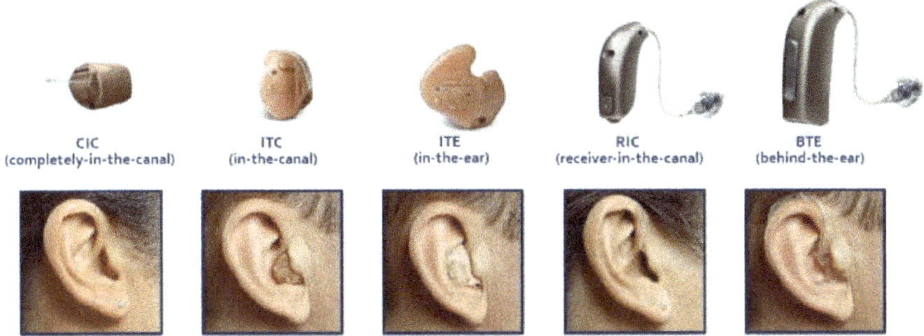

Fig. 9.1 Hearing aid types. Major variations of hearing aids include behind-the-ear (BTE), receiver-in-the-canal (RIC), in-the-ear (ITE), in-the-canal (ITC), and completely-in-the-canal (CIC) models.[3]

goals.[1] Moreover, hearing aid technology has grown increasingly convenient: hearing aids today are frequently equipped with Bluetooth capabilities to allow for hearing adjustments to be made via smartphone.[2] A few of the main types of present-day hearing aids are behind-the-ear (BTE) models, receiver-in-the-canal (RIC) models, in-the-ear (ITE) models, in-the-canal (ITC) models, and completely-in-the-canal (CIC) models (Figure 9.1).[1–3]

Each hearing aid model has unique features and indications. Likely the most recognizable of all hearing aid types, BTE hearing aids fit over the pinna and deliver sound through the external acoustic meatus to the cochlea for processing and recognition.[2] BTE hearing aids are indicated for patients with all ranges of hearing loss and all types of hearing loss, and they are considered the most powerful type of hearing aid.[2] BTE hearing aids are contraindicated if the hearing aids are unable to be placed appropriately due to other pathology or anatomical abnormality (aural atresia). BTE hearing aids can be more visible but are easy to use.[2] RIC hearing aids are a hybrid between BTE and ITE hearing aids: the microphone and processor are placed behind the ear, while the receiver sits in the ear canal to send acoustic signals to the tympanic membrane.[3] ITE hearing aids are a model of hearing aid where the receiver rests in the external acoustic meatus like a pair of wireless in-ear headphones.[2] ITE hearing aids are also indicated for hearing loss of all ranges and types.[2] ITE hearing aids are less visible than BTE hearing aids while retaining similar ease of use.[2] The third style of hearing aids, ITC hearing aids, are a less noticeable hearing aid option. Most of the device sits within the external auditory canal.[2] ITC hearing aids are indicated for mild-to-moderate hearing loss of any type.[2] ITC hearing aids are contraindicated in patients with severe-to-profound hearing loss.[2] Due to their placement location, ITC hearing aids are less visible and more difficult to adjust.[2] CIC hearing aids are placed entirely within the external auditory canal of the ear and are therefore nearly invisible.[2] Like ITC hearing aids, CIC hearing aids are indicated for mild-to-moderate hearing loss of all types and are contraindicated in patients with severe-to-profound hearing loss.[2] CIC hearing aids are considered more difficult to use and adjust and may not fit into all ear canals, given natural differences in anatomy of the ear.[2] Both ITC and CIC hearing aids should be placed by a medical professional. In addition to the aforementioned indications and contraindications of RIC, ITE, ITC, and CIC hearing aids, these devices are also contraindicated in settings where BTE hearing aids are contraindicated, as well as in patients with draining, wet ears, or in patients who have been surgically treated for a cholesteatoma with the canal wall down technique. All types of hearing aids are contraindicated if the patient lacks a fully developed cochlea or functioning cochlear nerve.

Regardless of the type utilized, hearing aids are an important treatment intervention in those with hearing loss and have been shown to provide favorable outcomes to patients. Hearing aids can also improve sentence recognition scores.[1] While outcomes are less successful in patients with severe-to-profound hearing loss, existing data indicate that appropriately selected and fitted hearing aids can assist patients in speech recognition both in quiet and in noise environments, although results varied widely in studies reviewed.[1] The reduced success in patients with severe-to-profound hearing loss and variation in results may be linked to the low signal-to-noise ratio that can hinder speech recognition in patients with severe-to-profound hearing loss.[1]

Bone-Anchored Hearing Aids

Bone-anchored hearing aids (BAHAs) are the first surgically placed devices discussed in this chapter. There is a small subset of bone conduction devices that are nonsurgically placed, most commonly indicated for children who cannot wear traditional hearing aids, such as aural atresia.[4] As an overview of the surgically implantable devices, BAHAs consist of an external sound processor and an internally placed screw, typically drilled into the mastoid process of the temporal bone. The sound processor collects sound from the environment, and sound vibrations cause the implanted screw to vibrate.[4] The cochlea picks up these vibrations, vibrating the fluid within the cochlea, stimulating the hair cells that transmit signals to the cochlear nerve, and sound is perceived.[4] BAHAs are indicated in children aged 5 years and older and adults and with mixed or conductive hearing loss. Both surgical and nonsurgical bone conduction devices are indicated for patients with unilateral or bilateral congenital atresia and unilateral or bilateral chronic ear disease with a conductive hearing loss or mixed hearing loss, which is refractory to treatment. BAHAs are not typically indicated in patients with purely sensorineural hearing loss because other treatment modalities — such as hearing aids or cochlear implants — are options more suited to target this type of hearing loss. BAHAs are contraindicated in patients with damage to the cochlea or portions of the cochlear nerve responsible for transfer of information between the cochlea and the cochlear nucleus in the brain. Soft contraindications for BAHA implantation include an extensive cranial surgery history due to poor suitable implantation site and a need for frequent MRIs to follow an intracranial pathology. The BAHA can cause a dense artifact onto the image, obscuring the temporal lobe anatomy. Healthcare providers should be aware of the risks and benefits of BAHAs when consulting patients on options to treat hearing loss and when following up with patients after procedures to treat hearing loss.

Among the bone conduction devices, there are surgical and nonsurgical passive transcutaneous types (Figure 9.2).[4] Among the surgical devices, there are two different types of BAHAs: percutaneous and transcutaneous (Figure 9.2).[4] Percutaneous BAHAs were the first developed BAHAs.[4] In percutaneous BAHAs, the implanted screw and external processor are connected through the skin.[4] Sound causes the external processor to vibrate, and these vibrations transmit directly to the implanted screw via their attachment.[4] The attachment, also known as the abutment, will become osseointegrated into the patient's bone.[4] The abutment transmits the vibration to the cochlea and the inner ear fluid, moving the hair cells and thereby stimulating the cochlear nerve.[4] This device is commonly stated as a "BAHA" although the formal name is Baha Connect (Cochlear). Given

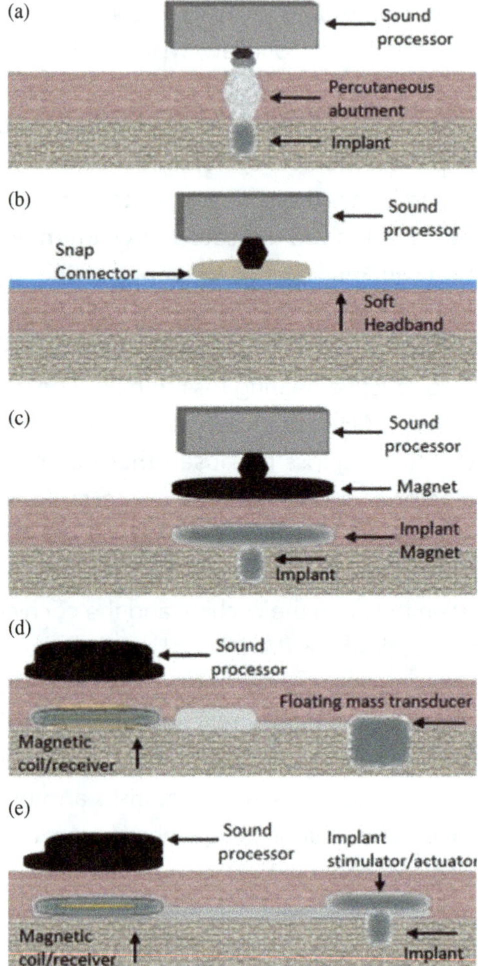

Fig. 9.2 The different types of bone conduction devices. **(a)** A surgical bone-anchored hearing aid (BAHA) that is percutaneous. **(b)** A nonsurgical bone conduction device that uses an adhesive or headband for this transcutaneous device. **(c)** A surgical BAHA that is passive transcutaneous using a magnet (BAHA Attract). **(d)** A surgical BAHA that is transcutaneous and active (Bonebridge). **(e)** A surgical BAHA that is transcutaneous and passive (Osia).[4]

the percutaneous connection between the abutment and the processor, adverse skin reactions such as infection and device extrusion can occur.[4] Adverse skin reactions are the most common complication with percutaneous BAHAs, and these adverse effects have caused this device to fall out of favor.[4] The second type of BAHA is the transcutaneous BAHA. The screw is still surgically placed in the mastoid under the skin, but unlike the percutaneous BAHA, the transcutaneous BAHA connects the internal and external components via magnets to fixate them, rather than piercing the skin for a physical connection.[4]

This manner of fixation reduces the issues that arise with infection and tissue regeneration that arises from piercing the skin.[4] However, transcutaneous BAHAs can still irritate the skin via the magnetic force applied to hold the device in place, and these devices are not as compatible with MRI as percutaneous BAHAs.[4] Percutaneous BAHAs are MRI compatible up to 3 Tesla, while transcutaneous BAHAs vary in MRI compatibility depending on the specific subtype, with most options being MRI compatible up to 1.5 Tesla and the Osia implant (see below) requiring removal of the internal magnet before proceeding with MRI.[4]

Further subdivision occurs in transcutaneous BAHAs, as two types exist: passive and active (Figure 9.3). In passive transcutaneous BAHAs, the external processor collects sound and vibrates, transmitting this vibrational energy from the processor to the screw through the skin.[4] There are two brands of passive transcutaneous BAHAs: Baha Attract (Cochlear) and the Sophono Alpha (Sophono Incorporated) (Figure 9.3). In active transcutaneous BAHAs, also known as active bone conduction implants, the external processor receives sound waves but does not vibrate.[4] Instead, it transforms this vibrational energy into electrical energy and sends an electrical signal to the implanted screw, and the screw then vibrates, transmitting energy through the bone to the cochlea, stimulating the cochlear nerve and enabling sound recognition.[4] There are two brands of active transcutaneous BAHAs, the Bonebridge (MED-EL) and the Osia (Cochlear) steady-state implant.

In the Bonebridge (BB) active conduction bone implant, the external processor collects environmental sounds and converts them into an electrical signal via a process called electromagnetic floating mass transducer.[4] This electrical signal is then sent to the internally implanted screw, which then vibrates.[4] The screw's vibrations cause the skull to vibrate, thereby the scala tympani and vestibuli fluid creating the same acoustic signal to the cochlea, enabling the perception of noise.[4]

The Osia steady-state active bone conduction implant operates in a very similar manner to the BB implant, but it is an osseointegrated implant and utilizes piezoelectric technology.[4] As an osseointegrated implant, the

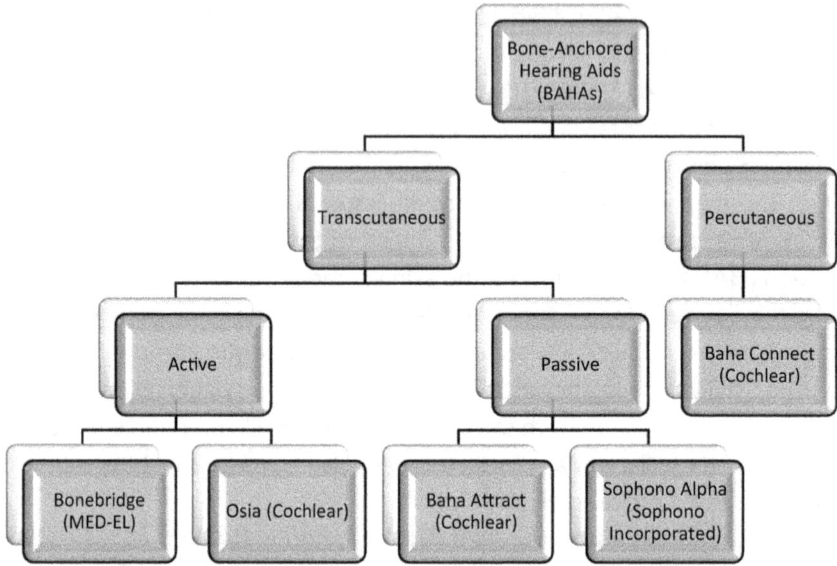

Fig. 9.3 Organizational tree of various types of surgical bone-anchored hearing aids (BAHAs). The two main classes of BAHA are transcutaneous and percutaneous BAHAs. Transcutaneous BAHAs can be subdivided into active and passive conduction devices.

Osia implant is completely fused with the bone and essentially becomes fully integrated into the skull.[4] Piezoelectric technology is the use of crystals to convert between mechanical energy and electrical energy, and this technology is used in the Osia implant to convert the vibrational energy of the sound waves that are collected via the external processor to an electrical signal which is sent to the osseointegrated implant.[4] This implant will then receive that signal and vibrate, causing the skull bones to vibrate and eventually stimulating the cochlea to allow for sound recognition.[4]

Both active, transcutaneous implantable devices (BB and Osia) are indicated in patients over the age of 5 years that have been diagnosed with mixed or conductive hearing loss and patients with single-sided deafness (SSD).[5] These devices are not considered a preferred treatment option in patients with sensorineural hearing loss and are contraindicated in patients with hearing deficits caused by retrocochlear lesions. This is because the purpose of these implantable devices is to provide another route for sound waves to travel and reach the cochlea, bypassing the outer and middle ear.

This alternative route is usually necessary in conductive or mixed hearing loss because the typical path sound waves take through the ear, through the middle ear, to the cochlea is altered. However, this alternative route does not help patients who have exclusively sensorineural hearing loss or retrocochlear pathology because the condition causing hearing loss is not bypassed by the alternative route.

Bone-anchored hearing aids are widely used, and outcomes are typically successful. Evidence shows implantation success rates of over 90% in multiple studies, although these success rates are lower in children and implant survival rates decline over time.[6] However, because transcutaneous BAHAs utilize magnets to fixate the processor and screw and do not pierce the skin permanently, these BAHAs may have less complications associated with skin and soft tissue.[6] Objective and patient-reported outcomes in both adults and children are favorable for BAHAs. In adults, BAHAs have been shown to improve free-field and sound-field thresholds in unaided and aided settings, and evidence demonstrates that they improve speech discrimination in quiet and noise when compared to previous users of conventional bone conduction hearing aids.[6] While the procedure is more complex in children for a variety of reasons, including but not limited to thinner temporal bones, outcomes are similar to those seen in adults.[6]

Cochlear Implants

Cochlear implants are surgically placed devices that consist of an internal magnet, antenna, and receiver/stimulator, which transmits the electrical signal through an electrode placed within the scala tympani and an external magnet, transmitter, processor, and microphone placed behind the ear.[7] Sound waves are collected by the external component and sent to the internal component as coded signals.[7] The internal component interprets these signals and sends electrical impulses to stimulate the spiral ganglion neurons in the cochlea, allowing the cochlear nerve to register and transfer sound information to the cochlear nucleus.[7] While patients can regain some sound awareness and speech perception with cochlear implants, the actual experience of hearing differs from people who do not use cochlear implants.

For the most part, cochlear implants are United States Food and Drug Administration (FDA) approved for adults and children >9 months with bilateral profound sensorineural hearing loss.[7] Cochlear implants are highly effective in both adults and children to provide sound awareness and open-set speech perception. Cochlear implants can also be used to treat tinnitus and auditory neuropathy spectrum disorder (ANSD). ANSD is predominantly a pediatric hearing disorder but can be seen in adults as well.[8] These are patients who may pass their newborn hearing screening, but have poor signaling upstream to the cochlea, and thereby have difficulty with pure tones and or speech.[8] Cochlear implants are not an ideal treatment option for patients with conductive hearing loss because other treatment options — like hearing aids and BAHAs — are more suitable. Contraindications to cochlear implant include a poorly developed cochlea and patients with retrocochlear pathology.[7] Additionally, cochlear implantation can be contraindicated when other conditions are present, such as active chronic otitis media or a ruptured tympanic membrane with active middle ear disease.[7] The path to success with a cochlear implant requires consistent and prolonged use in order to achieve open-set speech perception. However, if the patient cannot attend the numerous audiology appointments and or aural rehabilitation, then success with a cochlear implant is questionable. Another soft contraindication is intracranial pathology which may require continued imaging. Cochlear implant, while safe for CT and MRI, will cause a significant artifact, obscuring parts of the temporal lobe.

Cochlear implants present an exciting possibility for implant-based drug therapy. Combining medications with medical devices enables physicians to deliver prolonged, medical therapy to a localized area of body tissue and increase efficacy of implanted devices.[9] The use of stem cells to replace hair cell loss and gene therapy are other advancements that are anticipated with the cochlear implant.[9] A fully implantable cochlear implants represent another highly anticipated advancement in cochlear implant technology. These implants would be externally invisible, offering patients who wish to avoid any external signs of hearing loss a favorable option and potentially protecting the technology from external environmental trauma.

Auditory Brainstem Implants

The auditory brainstem implant (ABI) is a surgically placed implant that consists of an external microphone and processor placed behind the ear that collect sounds from the environment, a microchip transmitter placed just underneath the skin near the microphone and processor, and implanted electrodes that are placed on the brainstem (Figure 9.4). This is a more complex treatment, as the entirety of the afferent auditory tract is bypassed, and the dorsal cochlear nucleus is stimulated directly.[1] It requires a retrosigmoid or suboccipital craniotomy in order to access the auditory nucleus.[1]

Thus, this device is indicated in neurofibromatosis type 2 (NF-2) patients, patients with a defective or absent cochlea, patients with a damaged cochlear nerve, or patients in whom no other treatment is reasonable or successful.[10] Given the cochlear or retrocochlear nature of these pathologies, the ABI is the sole medical device indicated for treatment. The ABI is considered safe for use in both adult and pediatric populations. The FDA has approved it for patients ≥12 years old.[10]

Outcomes are mixed in adults and children fitted with ABIs, partially owing to the complexity of the pathophysiology involved. Adults have been shown to receive some auditory benefits from these implants, although some

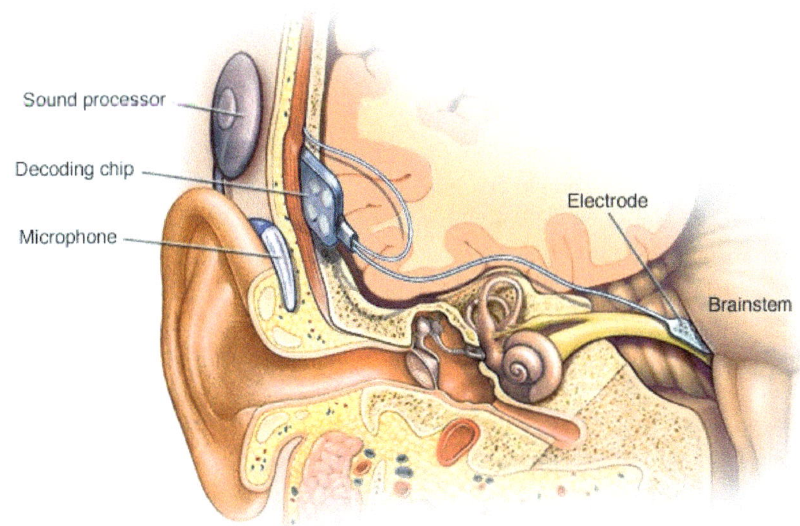

© MAYO FOUNDATION FOR MEDICAL EDUCATION AND RESEARCH. ALL RIGHTS RESERVED.

Fig. 9.4 Typical setup and pathway for an auditory brainstem implant.[10]

do not, and this must be considered along with the risks and benefits of any procedure.[10] In children, evidence indicates that ABIs can improve sound awareness albeit limited improvement in speech perception, although more research is required to confirm these findings and clarify which patients can benefit from ABIs and how much they can benefit.[10] At this time, ABIs are considered less successful than cochlear implants or other implantable devices to achieve the open-set speech understanding.[10] Cochlear implantation is generally preferred to auditory brainstem implantation in all potential patient populations without cochlear agenesis or retrocochlear pathology.

Conclusion

Medical devices can be used to treat patients with chronic hearing loss via a variety of mechanisms, all aimed at bypassing the damage to the auditory pathway that is impairing hearing. In this chapter, several classes of medical devices have been discussed, including hearing aids, BAHAs, cochlear implants, and ABIs. These devices vary in their function, uses, and invasiveness, so it is important that healthcare providers are capable of discussing the implications of each treatment option to tailor care to the individual needs of each patient.

References

1. National Research Council (US) Committee on Disability Determination for Individuals with Hearing Impairments. (2004) Sensory aids, devices, and prostheses. In: Dobie RA, Hemel SV, eds. *Hearing Loss: Determining Eligibility for Social Security Benefits*. Washington, DC: National Academies Press (US). Available at: https://www.ncbi.nlm.nih.gov/books/NBK207846/ (accessed September 6, 2022).
2. Nieman CL, Oh ES. (2020) Hearing loss. *Ann Intern Med* **173**(11):ITC81–96. doi:10.7326/AITC202012010.
3. Perfect Hearing. (2019) *Common Types and Styles of Hearing Aids*. Shah Alam: Perfect Hearing. Available at: https://perfecthearing.my/types-styles-hearing-aids/ (accessed September 6, 2022).
4. Snapp H. (2021) Bone conduction: Benefits and limitations of surgical and nonsurgical devices. *Otolaryngol Clin North Am* **54**(6):1205–17. doi:10.1016/j.otc.2021.07.015.

5. Cumpston E, Chen P. (2022) Implantable hearing devices. In: *StatPearls*. StatPearls Publishing. Available at: http://www.ncbi.nlm.nih.gov/books/NBK578178/ (accessed September 13, 2022).
6. Medical Advisory Secretariat. (2002) Bone anchored hearing aid: An evidence-based analysis. *Ont Health Technol Assess Ser* **2**(3):1–47. Available at: https://www.ncbi.nlm.nih.gov/pmc/articles/PMC3387772/ (accessed September 6, 2022).
7. United States Food and Drug Administration. (2020) *Nucleus 24 Cochlear Implant System — p970051/s172*. Silver Spring, MD: United States Food and Drug Administration. Available at: https://www.fda.gov/medical-devices/recently-approved-devices/nucleus-24-cochlear-implant-system-p970051s172 (accessed September 6, 2022).
8. Shearer AE, Hansen MR. (2019) Auditory synaptopathy, auditory neuropathy, and cochlear implantation. *Laryngoscope Investig Otolaryngol* **4**(4):429–40. doi:10.1002/lio2.288. PMID: 31453354; PMCID: PMC6703118.
9. Eshraghi AA, Nazarian R, Telischi FF, *et al.* (2012) The cochlear implant: Historical aspects and future prospects. *Anat Rec (Hoboken)* **295**(11):1967–80. doi:10.1002/ar.22580.
10. Deep NL, Roland JT Jr. (2020) Auditory brainstem implantation: Candidacy evaluation, operative technique, and outcomes. *Otolaryngol Clin North Am* **53**(1):103–13. doi:10.1016/j.otc.2019.09.005.

10 Cochlear Implants

Adrien A. Eshraghi, MD, MSc, FACS[1,2,3,4,5];
Maria-Pia Tuset, MD, MSc[1,5]; Jake Langlie, MD[1,5];
Thais Toledo, AuD,[1]; Meredith Holcomb, AuD,[1];
Mona Roshan, MS[1]; Fred F. Telischi, MD, MEE, FACS[1,2,3]

This chapter is dedicated to Dr. Thomas J. Balkany, MD, FACS, FAAP, who was a pioneer in cochlear implant surgery, a mentor and colleague to our team at the University of Miami Ear Institute.

Abstract

Cochlear implantation has emerged as the gold standard for severe-to-profound sensorineural hearing loss. The technological advances made in this field are continuously revolutionizing hearing rehabilitation. In this chapter, we will thoroughly discuss cochlear implantation. We will start with the pioneering discoveries that led to the cochlear implant (CI) and conclude with the current research in the field on the development of the optimal implant. We will discuss sound processing to understand the basic mechanisms of how CIs work and explain the implant characteristics and the main different types of implants available. As cochlear implantation criteria are

---

Corresponding Author: Adrien A. Eshraghi, MD, MSc, FACS

[1] Department of Otolaryngology, University of Miami Miller School of Medicine, Miami, FL, United States

[2] Department of Neurological Surgery, University of Miami Miller School of Medicine, Miami, FL, United States

[3] Department of Biomedical Engineering, University of Miami, Coral Gables, FL, United States

[4] Department of Pediatrics, University of Miami Miller School of Medicine, Miami, FL, United States

[5] Hearing Research and Cochlear Implant Laboratory, University of Miami, Miami, FL, United States

continuously expanding, we will also focus on demographics of CIs and current implantation criteria. Pre-operative evaluation and surgical approach are also explained to give a global view of the implantation process. Finally, the post-operative stages of implantation (programming, hearing rehabilitation), which are crucial in obtaining optimal hearing outcomes, are detailed along with the outcomes of implanted patients. This chapter aims to provide a comprehensive guide to cochlear implantation.

History of Cochlear Implants

Cochlear implants (CIs) are one of the major breakthroughs in the field of otology. Although they started to be available for use in patients with profound sensorineural hearing loss a little over 50 years ago, their development stemmed from the 1800s. The idea of electrical stimulation of the auditory system originated from Alessandro Volta, inventor of the electric battery in the early 1800s.[1] By inserting a metal probe connected to a battery in the external auditory canal, Volta was able to electrically transmit sounds with direct current, which he described as 'crackling, jerking or bubbling.'

Duchenne de Boulogne conducted some initial experiments and in 1855, Performed cochlear stimulation with alternating currents. This led not only to similar auditory sensations, but also to nonauditory stimulations such as metallic taste, most likely due to chorda tympani stimulation. The next breakthrough came in 1930. Electric potentials were recorded in the cochlea with waveforms closely matching the sound stimulus. This was termed the 'Wever and Bray effect' and brought about the possibility that hearing restoration could be achieved.[1]

The first direct electrical stimulation of the human auditory system, closest to current implant technology, was performed in 1957 by French electrophysiologist, André Djourno, and otolaryngologist, Charles Eyriès, on a patient having undergone numerous ear surgeries on both sides, where only the stump of the cochlear nerve remained. An electrode was placed in contact with the nerve and an induction coil with a ground electrode on the temporalis muscle. Electrical stimuli generated from a microphone were recorded, but only very poor discrimination was achieved, and the patient could not understand spoken speech.[1]

Dr. William F. House in Los Angeles is considered the first and foremost pioneer in cochlear implantation. Using the aforementioned work, he developed the first auditory prosthesis reliably used by patients. The first implants consisted of a single wire with a flamed ball contact at the tip or a five-electrode array. This innovation led to the first successful implantation in 1961. Dr. House, along with neurosurgeon Dr. John Doyle, developed a surgical approach allowing scala tympani insertion of the electrodes through the round window membrane, obtaining promising results. Patients were able to discriminate basic frequencies and identify words in small, closed sets. However, infection and electrode rejection required removal of the devices, and any further implantations were postponed. It was only later in 1967, when the first biocompatible devices were successfully implanted (pacemakers, ventriculoperitoneal shunts), that Dr. House and electrical engineer Jack Urban developed the first CI system safe enough to be used outside the laboratory environment. They collaborated with 3M Company and created the House/3M single channel device, making it the major landmark in the history of CI. Although large and heavy, they were the first to be worn by patients. Later developments gave rise to the multichannel CIs still used today.[1]

Cochlear implant was initially controversial, as the scientific community was largely critical of the invention, not believing that an implant would allow hearing restoration. This criticism was muted by a large study conducted by the National Institute of Health, which demonstrated that CI enabled important improvements in quality of life and significantly improved speech discrimination.

Support for CI grew immediately after, and over 1,000 patients were implanted from 1972 to the mid-80s, including several hundred children.[1] Although scientific approval was growing, and great progress in research was achieved, members of the deaf community argued that medical treatments of deafness threatened the deaf culture. Implantation was regarded as 'ethnocide,' or even unethical, and threatened efforts of the deaf community in regard to being members of a supportive ethnic group and not impaired or disabled. Time has passed, and CI has proved itself to be a safe and effective procedure. Its benefits leave minimal doubt that the procedure should be a standard choice for hearing rehabilitation in children and adults.

Demographics of CI Users and Current Indications for Implantation

According to a recent report on hearing from the World Health Organization, hearing loss is currently considered as the third largest cause of *years lived with disability* worldwide. Over 1.5 billion people live with hearing loss globally. This number is estimated to rise to 2.5 billion in the next 25 years. As of December 2019, approximately 736,900 CIs had been implanted worldwide.[2] In the United States, roughly 118,100 devices have been implanted in adults and 65,000 in children, representing only 24% of patients with severe-to-profound hearing loss in the United States. The U.S. Food and Drug Administration (FDA) first approved CI in adults in 1984 in post-lingually deafened adults aged 18 or older presenting with bilateral profound hearing loss (≥90 dB HL) and no speech recognition. Approval was then obtained in 1990 for children aged 2 years and older with profound bilateral hearing loss and no speech recognition.

Indications have progressively expanded in adults to include pre-lingually deafened adults and lower hearing thresholds (to moderate-to-profound hearing loss). Now, patients with significant residual hearing, which includes normal-to-moderate low frequency (<60 dB HL) or sloping to severe hearing loss (≥70 dB HL), with a speech perception of 10–60% in the ear may be candidates for surgery.[3] In children, current indications have lowered the age of implantation to less than 1 year of age in specific cases. Indications for early implantation also include severe-to-profound hearing loss and speech perception scores of <30% for open-set words.[3]

The most recent 2020 FDA change includes implantation of children as young as 9 months old and adds single-sided deafness and asymmetric hearing loss for patients aged 5 years or older with less than 10 years of deafness. This last addition is crucial as bone conduction hearing aids and contralateral routing of signals hearing aids were mainly used for these patients. These systems can deliver signals from the affected ear to the best hearing ear, but do not restore binaural signals contributing to sound localization or hearing speech in complex environments.

Most patients with sensorineural hearing loss also present with tinnitus coinciding with its varying levels of accompanying handicap. Clinicians started observing that tinnitus suppression was a common side effect of cochlear implantation in bilaterally implanted patients, which led to the development of several research protocols. There are many studies reporting the benefits of CI for patients with unilateral hearing loss for tinnitus suppression, with some studies even reporting improved speech recognition in noise and subjective reports of hearing benefit. A systematic review of literature recently reported that over 80% of patients with single-sided deafness and tinnitus experienced complete suppression or a decreased burden after implantation, but in 5% of patients, tinnitus worsened.[4] These results are creating increasing interest in patients with disabling tinnitus as common strategies for tinnitus treatment are often unsuccessful.

Another major development arose from the introduction of hybrid or electroacoustic devices (combination devices of a CI and a hearing aid in the same ear). In 2014, the FDA approved implantation of these devices for patients with significant residual hearing. Patients with profound high-frequency loss and significant residual low-frequency hearing still face social isolation with traditional hearing aids as this prevents from speech understanding in noisy conditions. Hybrid devices allow patients to integrate acoustic and electric signals and restore the consonant recognition necessary for users to unlock their residual low-frequency hearing. Outperformance of preoperative baselines in monosyllabic word recognition tests and music recognition tasks with and without lyrics have been achieved.

Common barriers to the use of hybrid devices seem to be the ability to preserve residual hearing over time. Some patients will experience discomfort coming from a lower signal-to-noise ratio tolerance with these types of implants and will eventually stop using acoustic stimulation and rely on pure electrical stimulation. Others will be driven by aesthetic concerns and physical discomfort from the additional acoustic part of the device. These challenges are currently the focus of many research centers to be overcome in the future.

An important factor to consider when expanding indications is the age at implantation in the older population. Hearing loss is a well-known factor in cognitive decline. Preservation of hearing can enhance social interactions and has been shown to delay the onset of dementia. In our practice, we have observed that even patients older than 80 years are candidates for implantation and have achieved significant benefits from CI.[5] Patient's comorbidities and risk factors must come into consideration when undergoing implantation under general anesthesia, but local anesthesia implantations have been safely performed and can be implemented in cases of severe comorbidities.

Sound Processing: How Do Cochlear Implants Work?

Cochlear implants are small, complex electronic devices that allow hearing restoration in patients with severe-to-profound hearing loss with an intact cochlear nerve by bypassing the damaged portions of the inner ear. The device consists of two parts: the external portion and a second internal, implanted part.

The external device has three components: a sound input unit (microphone, amplifiers, and filters) to capture sounds from the environment, a speech processor (digital signal processor) to select and arrange sounds picked up by the microphone, and a transmitter (radio-frequency link). The speech processor in the external unit extracts and encodes the spectral and temporal cues in speech and transmits this information to the internal unit. All these main components of the external unit are powered by a battery. The internal part consists of a magnet placed under the skin to communicate with the external portion of the implant. The device also contains a transmission system that transmits the converted electrical signal to the implanted electrode array surgically inserted into the scala tympani of the cochlea.

Another interesting function of the internal unit is to provide information to the user on the status of the electrodes. This is achieved by providing a back telemetry subunit. Signal transmission is performed transcutaneously through a radio frequency link using the principles of electromagnetic induction. The external transmitter encodes the stimulus information for radio-frequency transmission from the external coil to the implanted, internal coil. The internal receiver part then decodes the signal and stimulates the corresponding electrodes. The RF-link also serves to provide power to the internal unit for digital processing and current stimulation.[1]

The internal device has an electrode array that usually consists of multiple electrodes (from 12 to 22 depending on the implant brand) and stimulates the auditory nerve fibers in all regions of the cochlea (basal, middle, and apical regions). However, not all electrodes are stimulated simultaneously. The physiological cochlear tonotopy is used to transmit sound with basal electrodes being stimulated with high-frequency signals while apical electrodes are stimulated with low-frequency signals. The signal processor of a CI breaks the input signal into different frequency bands (or channels) and delivers the filtered signals to the appropriate electrodes. Signal processing techniques are developed to mimic the function of the healthy cochlea. The electrodes in the array will then stimulate the auditory nerve fibers in each cochlear region, and neural impulses will be propagated to the auditory processing pathways of the brain to be interpreted as sounds. The number of activated fibers is a function of the amplitude of the stimulus current. The loudness of the sound can be modulated by varying the amplitude of the stimulating current.

One of the most important features of an implant, and what differentiates implant brands, is the signal processing and current stimulation strategy. Each strategy used focuses on decoding and preserving main features of speech (waveform, envelope, and spectre). The fundamental strategies developed for signal processing are divided in two categories: waveform strategies and feature-extraction strategies. Waveform strategies present the waveform in an analogue or pulsatile form by filtering the speech signal into frequency bands. Feature extraction strategies present spectral features using feature extraction algorithms.

All modern sound processing strategies are based on the continuous interleaved sampling (CIS) strategy. This provides brief current pulses to each electrode such that no overlap occurs. The electric field interactions are minimized and allow for reduced power consumption. One of the main limitations in the CIS strategy is that it largely discards the temporal fine structure information of sound signal. Several strategies have derived from the CIS to overcome this issue, such as the fine structure processing strategy. Sound processing is one of the principal research areas in audiology with the goal of offering an individualized coding strategy in the near future.

Implant Characteristics: Focus on Electrode Design

For a CI user to fully benefit from their CI, the following factors need to be considered: (1) electrode array insertion depth and cochlear coverage, (2) matching neuro-tonotopicity, (3) atraumatic electrode array insertion and insertion forces against the intra cochlear structures, and (4) choice of an electrode array that matches the recipient's individual cochlear anatomy. The last is especially important when the patient's anatomy is malformed, and a regular CI electrode will not give an optimal placement close to the neural structures. A graphical representation of the normal anatomy of the inner, middle, and outer ear with cochlear implantation is provided in Figure 10.1.

Electrode array design is one of the main focuses in CI research.[6] Issues such as electrode placement, number, spacing, orientation, and configuration of electrodes are capital for optimal hearing outcomes. The

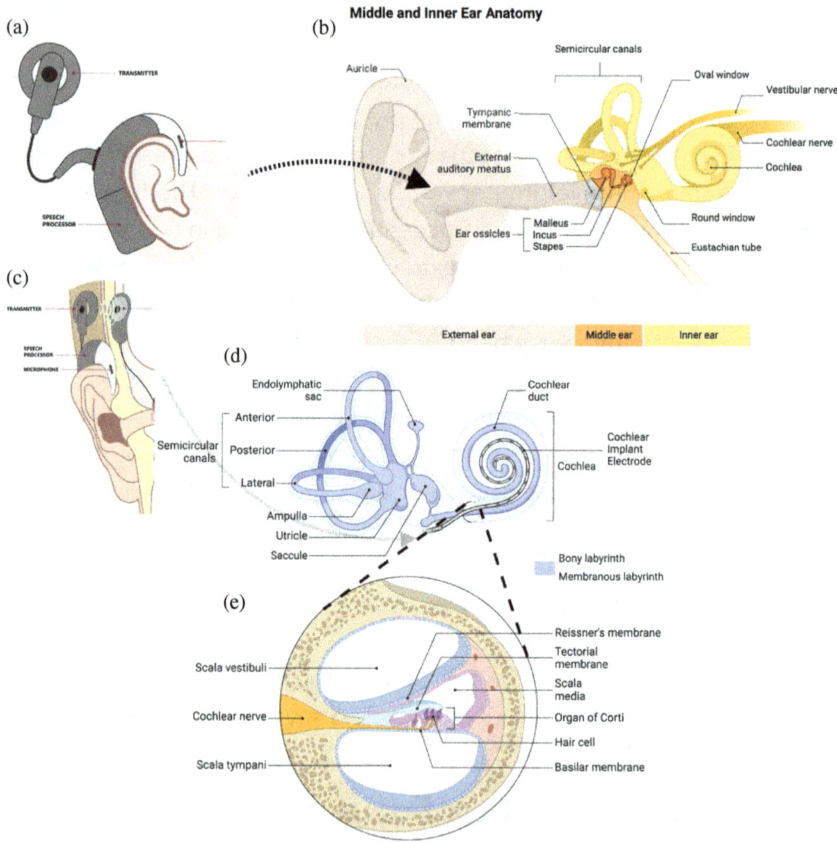

Fig 10.1 Outer, middle, and inner ear anatomy with cochlear implant (CI). **(a)** Diagram of the outer ear showing the speech processor, transmitter, and microphone of the CI. **(b)** Diagram demonstrating the anatomy of the external, middle, and inner ear. **(c)** Diagram representing the inner and outer portions. **(d)** Diagram representing the inner ear with a CI electrode. **(e)** Diagram depicting a cross-section of the cochlea. Diagram created using BioRender®.

electrode array is inserted in the cochlea through the round window or through a cochleostomy (drilled opening in the basal turn in proximity to the round window) and placed in the scala tympani when possible. Insertion depths usually range from 20 to 30 mm within the cochlea. The number of electrodes and spacing between affects the resolution for frequency coding. Two limiting factors in frequency coding exist: the number of surviving neurons and the spread of excitation associated from electrical stimulation. This fact is essential to provide high-definition electrical stimulation to the neural elements that cannot be fired through acoustic stimulation.

Two main types of electrode arrays are currently available. Straight arrays, also referred to as lateral wall arrays, lie along the lateral wall of the cochlea after placement. In contrast, perimodiolar arrays, or modiolus hugging arrays, have a curved preformed shape, which will place them near the modiolus. Several studies have shown that the use of a straight array creates less mechanical damage to the fragile sensory structures of the cochlea upon insertion, and so many institutions preferably use them for implantation in patients with greater residual preoperative hearing.[6,7]

Perimodiolar electrodes seem to require less electrical current to stimulate. Perimodiolar electrodes are also helpful in overcoming some of the complications of cochlear implantation, such as aberrant facial nerve stimulations, especially in patients presenting with temporal bone alterations as is the case of advanced otosclerosis. Some studies have demonstrated an increased risk of insertion trauma with their use due to the more rigid nature of the implant. The reported risk of electrode translocation for scala tympani to the scala vestibuli ranges from 26 to 40%, resulting in worse audiologic outcomes. To evaluate cochlear trauma, a grading system (ranging from 0 to 4) was established by Eshraghi *et al* in 2003 to better help assess electrode array trauma during insertion.[6] This has led to a better understanding of the degree of trauma caused by each electrode type, allowing surgeons to choose the right type of electrode in each specific case of cochlear implantation.

Pre-operative Evaluation of Patients

Pre-operative evaluation is always performed before CI surgery can be considered. Screening aims to select appropriate candidates and rule out those who do not meet the audiological criteria for CI or who have surgical contraindications.

The pre-operative screening may entail cognitive function tests or psychological evaluation when needed as well as meetings with CI audiologists. Together with the surgical team, appropriate assessment of CI candidacy is performed along with rehabilitation preparation.

Imaging is an essential part of the pre-implantation screening process. Usually, a computed tomography (CT)-scan and/or magnetic resonance imaging (MRI) is ordered by the surgeon and used to not only diagnose the cause of hearing loss, but also evaluate the anatomical considerations needed to perform the surgery safely and correctly. For instance, the presence of a cochlear nerve is essential for cochlear implantation, and confirmation of this via MRI is particularly important in pre-lingually deafened children who are CI candidates. In fact, the MRI is helpful in identifying the cochlear nerve, and full inner ear patency (absence of fibrosis), while the CT-scan only gives indirect signs of absence or presence via size of the internal auditory canal. CT-scans are also useful as they can indicate the patency of the cochlea (no ossification) and the presence of inner ear malformations, which can result in modifications of the surgical technique.

Another important point to consider is the anatomical position of the facial nerve in the middle ear. If the CI is placed incorrectly, the facial nerve may be at greater risk during surgery. Pre-operative CT-scans allow the surgical team to evaluate the necessary considerations for mastoid drilling, including pneumatization (presence of air) of the mastoid cavity with location of the sigmoid sinus and jugular bulb. When the mastoid cavity is particularly condensed and contracted, drilling is harder, and the chorda tympani may be sacrificed.

Absolute contraindications for cochlear implantation are cochlear nerve aplasia, absent cochlear nerve, and complete cochlear agenesis (absent cochlea). The remaining contraindications are relative and need to be considered on a case-by-case basis by a multidisciplinary committee involving a range of specialists (otologist, audiologist, radiologist, speech therapists, and psychologists). Patients presenting with significant intracochlear ossification or fibrosis, congenital malformations of the inner ear, or active chronic otitis must be carefully considered. Patients with psychiatric conditions that may result in an inability to use the CI or patients that lack motivation for the post-operative rehabilitation care must be carefully considered as implantation may not provide benefit.

A poor support system from family or friends is also a relative contraindication. Post-lingually deafened adults are currently contraindicated from cochlear implantation since the implant is not able to offer any speech recognition for these patients. However, they may benefit from environmental warning sounds for their safety (traffic noise, alarms). CI may be discussed with the different members of the implantation team. Appropriate expectations should be thoroughly discussed and understood by the patient prior to implantation.

Surgical Approach for Cochlear Implantation

Cochlear implantation is performed under general anesthesia with the patient typically returning home after a few hours of surveillance following surgery. An overview of the steps of the surgery is provided in Figure 10.2.

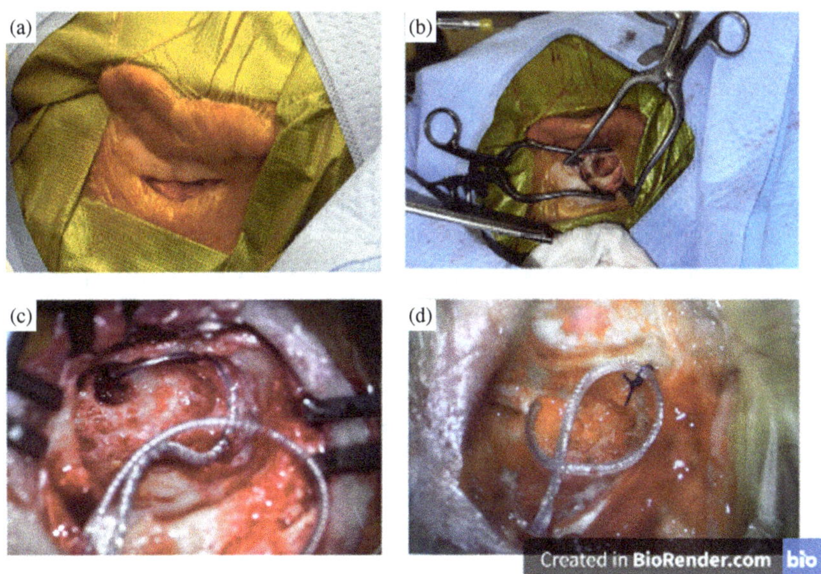

Fig 10.2 Images of Right Cochlear Implant Surgery Steps. **(a)** Incision of the retro-auricular skin. **(b)** Mastoidectomy is performed, the temporalis flap is prepared prior to cochlear implantation. **(c)** The internal device is placed in the temporalis pocket and the cochlear implant electrode is inserted fully into the cochlear turns through the round window membrane. **(d)** The electrode is secured in round window and facial recess by temporal fascia and muscle grafts, the electrodes secured in mastoid cavity with a proline suture.

Every surgeon and surgical Center has their own techniques, but the main steps for implantation are similar in cases of standard cochlear implantation. Surgical steps have been refined over time with smaller incisions and soft surgical techniques which strive to minimize inner ear damage.

After induction of general anesthesia, intraoperative facial nerve monitoring is prepared by placing subcutaneous needle electrodes in the patient's face on the operated side. The monitoring uses electromyography to monitor the response of facial muscles. Electrodes will be placed 10–15 mm externally to the superior eyelid (orbicularis oculi muscle) and 10–15 mm externally to the corner of the mouth (orbicularis oris muscle). This process of monitoring the facial nerve ensures an additional safety measure to prevent trauma to the facial nerve. The surgical area, consisting of the ear and surrounding area, is disinfected using the appropriate aseptic protocols applied in each operation room (iodine or chlorhexidine solution application for most cases). A local anesthetic is injected post auricularly in the incision area, and the surgical microscope will be placed in front of the patient.

A post-auricular incision is performed 3–5 mm behind the post-auricular crease. An anterior periosteal flap centered around the external auditory canal is elevated in a U-shape to expose the temporal bone and identify the bony landmarks of the posterior external auditory canal. This step creates a tight pocket to house the receiver-stimulator in the superior part of the temporalis muscle incision (Balkany Receiver-Stimulator Pocket). This is an important step as device migration is a known post-operative complication, which can lead to interference with the external processor, wound complications, device extrusion, or even device failure.

The long-standing method for fixation of the device is to create a bony well seat for the shape of the receiver-stimulator. If drilling is performed, caution and care are emphasized to avoid the dural membrane, especially in children where skull thickness is only 2–3 mm. As CI evolves towards thinner designs, the need for implant bed drilling disappears, and a tight temporalis pocket between the temporal-parietal and lambdoid sutures (Balkany Pocket) is enough for secure fixation with comparable migration and operative times.

After securing the receiver-stimulator, a mastoidectomy is performed. During this procedure, the surgeon drills into the mastoid cavity, a part of the temporal bone, to allow access into the middle and inner ear. Drilling is continued until the mastoid antrum and all lateral mastoid air cells are removed. The lateral semicircular canal is exposed and constitutes a useful landmark, along with the incus, for the facial nerve position. The facial recess, a triangular region delineated superiorly by the fossa incudes (incus), facial nerve posteriorly, and chorda tympani anteriorly, can now be identified. A posterior tympanotomy is then performed, referring to the wide opening of the facial recess. This step is essential as the inferior portion of the facial recess allows visualization of the round window niche. The facial recess is usually already of adult size at birth, which is important when implanting children under 12 months old. It is very important to analyze the facial nerve position as abnormal nerves are often associated with malformations of the inner ear, such as common cavity anomalies or semicircular canals anomalies, where the nerve passes on top of the cochlea and is sometimes split.

After opening the facial recess and obtaining wide visualization of the round window niche, the cochlea can be approached. One of the following techniques is usually used for electrode insertion in the scala tympani: round window insertion, extended round window approach, or a cochleostomy approach. When the round window membrane is properly visualized and favorably oriented, it can be incised, and the electrode implanted directly through. In some cases, the bony overhang of the round window hides the round window membrane and needs to be drilled at a decreased speed. This technique allows for ideal intracochlear placement through the round window membrane. If the round window insertion is not possible, cochleostomy is performed, consisting of drilling the basal turn anteriorly and inferiorly to the round window using a 0.6–1 mm diamond burr at decreased drilling speed. This area allows electrode insertion at the same level as the scala tympani floor. Some surgical teams advocate for hyaluronic acid application after the cochlea has been opened to limit perilymph loss. Perilymph suction is avoided at all costs to avoid inner ear trauma, especially in cases where hearing preservation is desired.

Electrode insertion in the scala tympani is usually the last step of the surgery to minimize potential trauma to the inner ear. The tip of the electrode array is directed anteriorly and inferiorly to ensure complete atraumatic insertion into the scala tympani. Insertion is conducted slowly and smoothly by the surgeon, stopping at the first point of resistance. Over-insertion may result in electrode tip fold-over leading to degraded speech perception results. Cochleostomy or round window opening is sealed by fascia and helps to stabilize the electrode, prevent extrusion, and limit possible infections of the inner ear or meninges. Each manufacturer recommends a specific insertion technique with their electrodes and surgeons need to be familiar with each electrode type and brand they use. The electrode is secured in the facial recess with a muscle graft.

After insertion, the periosteal flap is closed. The stimulator-receiver and electrode leads are covered to prevent any device extrusion. Resorbable sutures are used to suture subcutaneous tissues. The skin may be closed with resorbable sutures.

Although intra-operative monitoring is performed in many centers to confirm device integrity and appropriate electrode placement, it is not a standardized procedure. This testing involves implant impedance testing and neural response telemetry testing and is dependent upon the implant brand used. These results may be useful for the implant programming. Each manufacturer provides the intraoperative testing devices. Immediate post-operative X-ray or CT-scans are performed by some teams to confirm intracochlear electrode placement and rule out any tip fold-over or electrode extrusion, particularly in cases of inner ear malformation or specific electrode designs (i.e., perimodiolar).

Rehabilitation After CI and Programming

After surgical insertion of the CI, patients usually wait one month for the implantation site to heal. After healing of the surgical site, activation of the implant and use of the external processor can begin. Appointments typically follow a pre-set schedule at: 1-week post-operative, 1-month follow-up for initial stimulation, the following 3 months for appropriate mapping, and continuous programming sessions ranging from 6 to 12 months for the duration of implant use.

Once the CI is activated, sound can be heard but may not be understood by the patient initially. Intensive auditory rehabilitation is necessary to attach meaning to the new signals produced by the CI. Some teams, however, have described successful activations as early as day 1 post-operative, although this is not common practice. Initial activation of the CI typically occurs 2–4 weeks after CI surgery.[8] The goal of this appointment is to provide audibility to the patient by setting the CI upper stimulation levels to a comfortable volume. Patients should be able to detect sounds in their environment but are not necessarily expected to understand speech on the day of activation.

Following activation, the patient is expected to return 3–4 times during the first year of CI use for programming/mapping visits. During the mapping process, a combination of objective data collected from the implant and the patient's individual subjective perception of sound quality are used for fine-tuning the CI. Throughout these visits, the audiologist will work to provide the patient with appropriate access to sounds in the near-normal hearing range with the goal of improving speech understanding. Post-operative testing is also performed at various visit intervals in the sound booth to track the patient's speech perception progress with the CI. Adjustments for sound quality are performed as the patient's speech perception with the CI improves.

Cochlear implant programming, the adjustment of the external processor based on the auditory perception of the electrical stimuli provided by the implant, continues over the life of the implant. This plan is tailored to the patient and the implant. During the initial programming sessions, auditory information is not able to be processed fully as the cranial nerves and brain are acclimating to the use of the implant. As the brain continues to adjust to the implant stimulation, patients will begin to have significant improvement in understanding speech over the following 6 months after implantation. Continuous programming sessions are essential to refine and adjust stimulation of the auditory nerve for optimal auditory outcomes.

One of the most important factors of CI rehabilitation is daily device use. Patients should wear the CI processor a minimum of 11 hours per day to optimize their overall speech understanding performance.[9] This allows time for the brain to adapt to the new information it is now receiving, and to provide the brain with consistent input. Over time, the brain learns to interpret this new information into usable speech and the patient's speech perception with the CI improves.

Listening practice, listening through only the CI, is also crucial to the patient's progress with the implant. Streaming information from a smartphone or tablet is one recommended method to complete listening practice. Listening rehabilitation apps, audiobooks, and podcasts provide self-directed practice to improve speech perception through the patient's CI. One-on-one speech therapy sessions with a speech pathologist is another method available for adult CI users.

To achieve the best outcomes, the patient, audiologist, and auditory rehabilitation team work together throughout the life of the implant to continually check hearing outcomes and adjust programming of the implant. Additional services, including speech therapy, may be provided to the patient to help in auditory therapy, especially in cases of pediatric implantations. The length and duration of these appointments will vary as the patient's brain works to understand and interpret stimulation from the CI.

In contrast to adults who have previously developed language skills prior to implantation, pre-lingual children who have not yet begun speaking must develop their language skills concurrently with the use of the CI. In addition to regular follow-up of the implant, children often undergo weekly auditory or speech rehabilitation sessions to enhance and track auditory outcomes. Children are known to have enhanced neuroplasticity, or the brain's ability to modify and change in response to experiences. These sessions take advantage of this concept to improve auditory outcomes. However, adults and children both require an auditory stimulating environment post-implantation to enhance hearing outcomes.

While rehabilitation in adults is defined as an intervention for patients who are understanding to hear again, habilitation in children is defined as an intervention for patients who have not heard before. Both are essential components of care following implantation. To perform rehabilitation of hearing, speech language pathologists, audiologists, and otologists work together to create an individualized care plan, addressing the needs of communication management, auditory therapy, and adjustment to the patient's new auditory environment. Each rehabilitation program works methodically to develop, imitate, and associate meaning of the patient's auditory environment to spoken language. During CI rehabilitation, guidance and specialized strategies are used to enhance interpretation of auditory stimulation and encourage goal-based therapy.

Outcomes of Cochlear Implantation

Quality of life

Quality of life following cochlear implantation has been shown to significantly improve, based on the concept that hearing allows greater engagement and interaction with one's environment. Although it can be expected that adult patients will not achieve the same outcomes post-implantation that they experienced prior to the onset of hearing loss, significant gains in hearing and interpretation of vocal emotions have been shown to enhance a patient's quality of life.

It has been shown that following implantation adults have greater independence, more occupational opportunities with higher skills positions, improved communication and socialization, greater well-being, and decreased depressive symptoms.[5] In children, development of language and early inclusion in neurotypical school system is achieved. Although there are currently no measures to predict how an individual's quality of life will improve following cochlear implantation, it can be expected that most individuals will have an increase in overall well-being and quality of life. However, there is a need for families and professionals to continue to support the implant recipient and help the individual cope with gaps between actual and expected hearing outcomes as they adjust to the use of the implant.

Continual encouragement of individuals following implantation provides a supportive and empowering experience for the user. Although individuals may experience improvement in quality of life within the first year of use, it is important to counsel patients that the more years a patient uses their implant, the greater the benefits and quality of life they will achieve. It has been shown that there is a correlation between gain of speech perception and quality of life with individuals rating an increase in their quality of life as their hearing improves.

Music Perception

The full spectrum of auditory perception required to appreciate the tones, pitch, and quality of music is one of the more difficult skills to achieve following implantation. Given the limited number of electrodes in a CI, it can be difficult to convey all qualities of the frequency and intensities present in music. As music perception has been shown to be a factor in improvement of quality of life, the field is an ongoing area of research to improve implantation outcomes.

There are many factors that are known to impact the ability to enjoy music following implantation. Among these include musical education, age at implantation, and lived experiences of the patient. It is important to counsel patients on the expected outcomes prior to implantation and to understand their prior level of musical education. If playing or listening to music played an important component of the patient's life prior to implantation, there are specific programs of music acquisition following implantation that the patient can pursue. Although individuals may not have the same ability to listen to music following implantation, there is still a gain of hearing that translates into increased enjoyment brought from song.

Enjoying music with a CI requires the individual to identify the harmonic and melodic components of music that constitute a song. Situations of a large ensemble or orchestra can be a point of frustration during the first few years following implantation. Therefore, it is recommended to start by listening to simple, nonlyrical pieces that you are familiar with in the past. Simple pieces, composed of only a few instruments, can allow the user to learn how to utilize their implant so, eventually they may listen to all components of the piece. It is suggested to counsel patients on listening to songs with clear pronunciation early on. As the individual starts to become comfortable, they can begin to introduce more complex pieces, including multiple vocalists, instruments, and tempos.

Although music perception may be different to the typical CI user following implantation, individuals should not be discouraged by their progress, but instead, reminded that with time and practice, they will enjoy the complex rhythms and tempos of music.

Hearing Preservation in Cochlear Implantation

Cochlear implants were designed to bypass the middle and inner ear structures and directly stimulate the cochlear nerve. Implanted patients initially have bilateral, severe-to-profound sensorineural hearing loss across all frequencies and no word recognition upon speech testing. Continuous advances in cochlear implantation technology, such as sound processing and surgical techniques, have allowed for improved hearing outcomes in patients.[10,11] These improvements have permitted criteria for cochlear implantation to progressively expand and include patients with more residual hearing. When patients with residual hearing can be implanted, preserving the remaining functional structures of the patient's inner ear is essential. In most cases, patients will experience high-frequency hearing loss, corresponding to the frequency range covered by the basal turn of the cochlea, but may still have residual hearing in the low frequencies that are covered by the middle and apical regions of the cochlea. It is estimated that 72–85% of cochlear implantation candidates have aidable bilateral low-frequency residual hearing before surgery with this number increasing steadily over time.[12]

Cochlear implantation of patients with significant functional residual hearing allows for the use of a hybrid or electroacoustic device. These devices combine the CI for the stimulation of high frequencies and a hearing aid to use the residual functional frequencies in the cochlea. Patients implanted with electroacoustic devices have demonstrated improved speech perception in noise, improved sound localization, and music appreciation.

Several techniques have been described to achieve better hearing preservation. 'Soft surgery' techniques have been developed to minimize trauma to the fragile inner ear structure during electrode array insertion. Performing insertion through a cochleostomy or a round window approach is one of the main factors that was evaluated for these techniques. Many teams have found round window insertion to cause less trauma to the inner ear including organ of Corti preservation and lower rates of electrode translocations.[13] Slow and controlled electrode advancement during implantation has been shown to achieve better rates of successful post-operative hearing results with the development of further improvement expected with robotic-assisted insertion underway.

Electrode design has been a focus for hearing preservation. Initially, the surgical technique relied on partial electrode insertion or on the use of shorter electrodes to avoid damage to the apical regions of the cochlea.[7] CI manufacturers have been intensely focused on developing softer, thinner, and more flexible arrays to minimize trauma. A grading system of ear trauma post electrode insertion has been developed by our team and is now widely used by researchers and physicians around the globe.[6]

While perimodiolar electrodes have emerged to provide great hearing outcomes, their modiolus-hugging shape has been shown to increase the rate of scalar translocations (grade 3 or 4 inner ear trauma according to the Eshraghi and Balkany grading system), with a higher percentage of scala vestibuli insertions compared to lateral wall. Figure 10.3 depicts perimodiolar versus lateral wall electrodes positioning inside the cochlea. These translocations lead to increased traumatic reactions to the inner ear structures and create not only an immediate, but also a delayed inflammatory reaction affecting cochlear anatomy and may lead to increased intracochlear fibrosis and possible ossification. Figure 10.4 depicts a graphical representation of trauma to the inner ear during insertion and provides the grading system that describes the severity of the inner ear trauma.

To improve hearing protection and manage the inflammatory reactions caused by cochlear implantation, pharmacologic therapies can also be

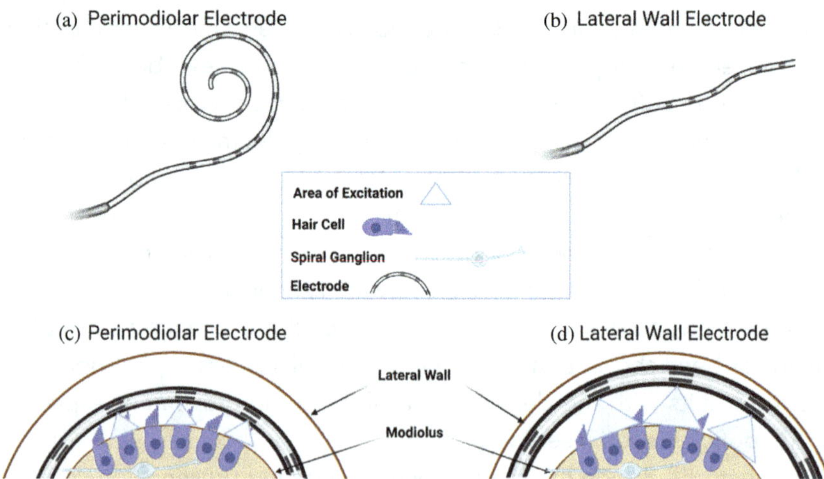

Fig 10.3 Electrode types and positioning. **(a)** Graphical representation of a perimodiolar electrode. **(b)** Graphical representation of a lateral wall electrode. **(c)** Diagram demonstrating the area of excitation of the residual hair cells and spiral ganglion cells of a perimodiolar electrode. **(d)** Diagram demonstrating the area of excitation of the residual hair cells and spiral ganglion cells of a lateral wall electrode. Diagram created using BioRender®.

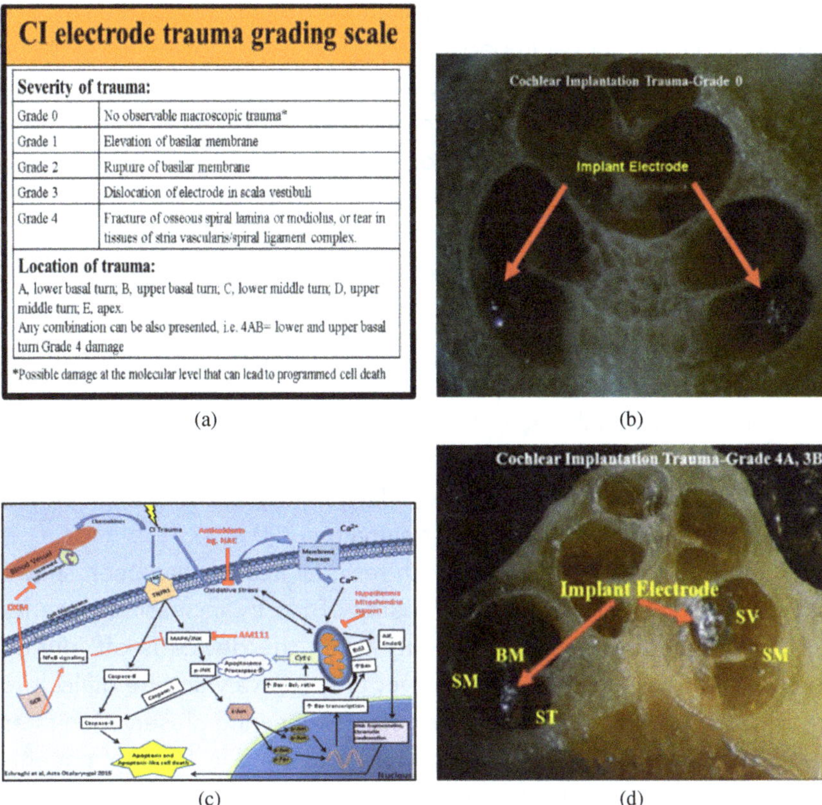

CI electrode trauma grading scale

Severity of trauma:	
Grade 0	No observable macroscopic trauma*
Grade 1	Elevation of basilar membrane
Grade 2	Rupture of basilar membrane
Grade 3	Dislocation of electrode in scala vestibuli
Grade 4	Fracture of osseous spiral lamina or modiolus, or tear in tissues of stria vascularis/spiral ligament complex.

Location of trauma:

A, lower basal turn; B, upper basal turn; C, lower middle turn; D, upper middle turn; E, apex.
Any combination can be also presented, i.e. 4AB= lower and upper basal turn Grade 4 damage

*Possible damage at the molecular level that can lead to programmed cell death

Fig 10.4 Inner ear trauma figures and scale (Eshraghi and Balkany inner ear trauma scale). **(a)** Cochlear implant (CI) electrode trauma grading scale. **(b)** Representative image of cochlear implantation trauma grade 0 indicating no observable macroscopic damage to the cochlea during insertion. **(c)** Graphical representation of the molecular mechanisms underlying inflammation and apoptosis of hair cells following electrode insertion trauma. Diagram created using BioRender® and some proposed therapeutics in red. **(d)** Representative image of cochlear implantation trauma grade 4A, 3B depicting fracture of osseous spiral lamina at the lower basal turn and dislocation of the electrode into Scala vestibuli at the upper basal turn respectively.

used.[14,15] Glucocorticoids are steroid molecules commonly used to reduce inflammatory reactions. These molecules are used orally by many surgeons teams during the perioperative period yet no proven efficacy on residual hearing preservation has been found during clinical trials. Electrode arrays coated with glucocorticoids are also being developed and investigated as they provide extended steroid release to the cochlea with higher concentrations.[16] These electrodes have shown great promise with ongoing clinical trials in Europe showing preliminary success in hearing preservation and keeping the inner ear impedance lower (indirect sign of intracochlear fibrosis or ossification). Several molecules with diverse action patterns are being evaluated for hearing preservation at this time. Drug-delivery systems to the inner ear are an important area of research as they lead to hearing preservation, and therefore, can help to expand the indication of CI to patients with more residual hearing.

Data suggest that the best audiologic hearing preservation outcomes are most consistently achieved with a round window approach, slow insertion speed, and local and systemic glucocorticoid administration. A systematic review of published scientific papers analyzed over 650 implants inserted by various international surgeons. Comparisons between the various types of electrodes all using the Eshraghi/Balkany grading system demonstrated radiological and histological evidence of lateral wall electrodes having lower inner ear trauma (Eshraghi/Balkany trauma grade 0 or 1).[17]

Overall, implanting patients with residual hearing has been shown to provide significant benefits on quality of life by increasing patient's self-confidence and sense of security when the device is off (during sleep, swimming). However, results over time can vary and be difficult to predict. A study evaluating long-term residual hearing preservation rates found that although residual hearing was preserved in 100% of patients immediately post-operatively, only 25% of patients had complete residual hearing preservation at 24-months, and 12.5% had complete loss of residual hearing.[18] Development of intra-operative monitoring of the cochlear electrophysiological characteristics has emerged as a useful tool to predict surgical outcomes on residual hearing preservation. Using the CI electrodes, electrocochleography can be performed to measure acoustically evoked potentials and evaluate the cochlear auditory function post-implantation.

While inner ear structure and hearing preservation is currently one of the main focuses of research on cochlear implantation as it provides great benefits for patients as it was mentioned previously, it also provides an opportunity for possible application of future advances of research such as gene therapy or regenerative medicine. Advances in imaging technology such as OTOPLAN® also help in selecting individualized electrode for each patient based on the accurate size of their inner ear cochlea. OTOPLAN features automatic pre-op cochlear parameter measurements[19] and electrode visualization in post-op. It also allows a more personalized medicine with anatomy-based fitting aiming to avoid electrode cochlear frequency mismatch. The device has been demonstrated to provide accurate reconstructions of the full inner ear including the cochlea, round window membrane, bony overhang, semi-circular canals, and internal auditory canal and detect possible inner ear malformations. The software can fuse both MRI and CT scans, allowing the most accurate preview of the insertion depth.[20,21]

Ongoing Research Perspectives

Otoprotection in Cochlear Implantation

Electrode array insertion into the cochlea leads to structural damage to the cochlea but concurrently triggers an inflammatory reaction at the time of insertion.[22] This inflammatory reaction is immediate and starts after implantation. In addition, the presence of a foreign body in the cochlea can also lead to a chronic inflammatory reaction and eventually, cochlear fibrosis. To protect the auditory system, a wide range of drugs have been tested to protect the auditory system by counteracting the inflammatory reactions triggered by the procedure.[14,15] Steroids (such as dexamethasone) have been particularly studied for their anti-inflammatory properties, but antioxidants (N-acetylcysteine), growth factors (neurotrophins), and immunosuppressants (TNF-α, IFN) have also been tested. Neurotrophins are particularly interesting as they promote neural tissue regrowth and are involved in neuronal health throughout life. Some of the neurotrophic growth factors can regenerate peripheral nerve fibers and stop spiral ganglion cell degeneration.

Local drug delivery to the cochlea has been shown to be an effective method of application, resulting in fewer side effects compared to systemic (oral or intravenous) administration. Efficient inner ear delivery systems are actively researched, and one of these systems includes using the CI itself. CIs coupled with osmotic mini pumps allowing sustained drug delivery have been widely tested but pose the disadvantage of being prone to infection and restricted patient usability. As an alternative to minipump delivery, drug-eluting electrodes have been developed. These electrodes are coated with a drug that will be slowly released in the inner ear. The advantage of this system is that the electrode itself is used, however the diffusion of the drug over time can be difficult to estimate and manage. These devices hold much promise for the future. Research on this field is continuously expanding, and clinical trials focusing on safety and tolerance of otoprotective drugs are emerging.

Robotic Surgery

Surgical technique for cochlear implantation is a standardized procedure, and most research teams have focused their efforts on other domains (drug therapy, electrode design) to improve CI outcomes. However, this approach has changed since robotic systems and image-guided surgeries have emerged in many surgical fields as a revolutionary utility. They allow for more precise and controlled movements, work in confined spaces, and allow for minimally invasive approaches.[23] The technology has proved to be useful in neurotology, particularly during cochlear implantation. Robots are currently being tested clinically in different surgical steps of implantation.

Using three-dimensional (3D) CT, temporal bone drilling can be planned and programed by the robot to avoid all sensible structures. Automated robots have the advantage of drilling into areas invisible to the surgeon and can avoid excessive exposure of the mastoid, often necessary in cochlear implantation and other neurotological procedures. Additionally, they have pre-programed drilling depths to avoid damage to crucial anatomical landmarks, such as the facial nerve, the dura, or venous structures.[23] Efforts on robotic CI surgery have focused on creating industrial robotic manipulators, surgical templates for guided keyhole drilling of the mastoid, bone attachments of the robot, image-based surgical planning, robotic electrode insertion systems, and robotic drilling force-feedback control. Several centers are conducting successful clinical trials using robot-assisted cochlear implantations.[23,24] As previously discussed, residual hearing preservation is a priority in cochlear implantation, and a robot-assisted electrode insertion has been proved to better control the angle and speed of insertion, decreasing inner ear trauma.

Optical Cochlear Implant

Electrical stimulation of the auditory nerve is the basis of current CI technology. However, electrical current can be hard to focus in conductive environments, such as the cochlea, impacting quality of hearing. Optical stimulation of the auditory neurons has emerged as an interesting alternative to this issue.[25,26] Photonic stimulation of hair cells or spiral ganglion neuron cells could improve the dynamic range of stimulation, allowing patients to have a better understanding of speech in noisy environments and increased music appreciation. To achieve this, two main stimulation strategies have been explored: infrared laser stimulation and optogenetic stimulation. Infrared neural stimulation uses an implanted laser device to stimulate neurons through heat. The main challenge of this technique is creating efficient neural stimulation without damaging the cells. A more complex, but promising, approach seems to be optogenetic stimulation, which uses both gene therapy technology through transfection of cells using viral vectors (viruses engineered to carry and transfer genes to human cells) and optical stimulation by implanting an optical fiber in the cochlea.[25] Since light is conveniently confined in space, it is speculated that smaller tonotopic ranges can be activated by this type of stimulation, increasing the quality of encoded sound. This translates into a greater number of electrodes in the array. Neurons will be transfected with genes, making them photosensitive. Although promising in theory, this technology is still a long way from clinical translation.

Towards a Customized Cochlear Implant

One of the main goals of cochlear implantation is to restore quality hearing in as many patients as possible. With the expansion of CI candidacy, patients with inner ear malformations have been included, highlighting the need for customized electrode designs matching the patient's anatomy. With the emergence of 3D printing technologies and high-resolution 3D CT-scans, manufacturers are aiming to provide the optimal electrode for the patient's unique anatomy. These electrodes, combined with the appropriate pharmaceutical, genetic, or cellular treatment target for the patient, could provide ideal custom-made CI electrodes. Currently, simple measures such as electrode array length matched to cochlear length are already considered when implanting patients and are becoming standard practice in many centers.

Another important consideration in improving cochlear implantation in patients is developing a fully implantable CI. This has been a major goal for manufacturers as it would provide patients with the ability to continuously hear in any environment (wet, dust). Other important advantages include reduced wear and tear and a fully invisible implant, which may reduce the stigma experienced by the patient. Although trials of fully implantable devices have been successfully conducted, there are still many challenges before clinical implementation can begin.

Cochlear Implants of the Future

With all these developments underway, there are still many challenges and opportunities in the field of cochlear implantation. We can imagine new charging technologies for CIs, with increased battery duration, or the possibility of durable charging techniques, such as solar charging. Additionally, implants may be improved to be not only fully MRI compatible, but also able to reduce artefact upon imaging. The future CI may be smaller and fully implantable, eliminating the social stigma some patients fear and experience. Designing an implant with an internal device that can be changed without the need to remove the electrode array from the cochlea would also be a groundbreaking development, allowing for easier upgrade or replacement of the internal device in case of failure. Further development of remote programming and fitting of CIs would increase patient comfort as they would not need to travel frequently to implant centers. Finally, with technological developments in robotic surgery, remote surgery may become an option in the future, allowing patients with limited access to specialized surgeons to undergo cochlear implantation in their nearest hospital.

References

1. Eshraghi AA, Nazarian R, Telischi FF, *et al.* (2012) The cochlear implant: Historical aspects and future prospects. *Anat Rec (Hoboken)* **295**(11):1967–80.

2. World Health Organization. (2021) World report on hearing. World Health Organization.
3. Krogmann RJ, Al Khalili Y. (2022) *Cochlear Implants*. In: *StatPearls* [Internet]. Treasure Island, FL: StatPearls Publishing.
4. Peter N, Liyanage N, Pfiffner F, *et al.* (2019) The influence of cochlear implantation on tinnitus in patients with single-sided deafness: A systematic review. *Otolaryngol Head Neck Surg* **161**(4):576–88.
5. Eshraghi AA, Rodriguez M, Balkany TJ, *et al.* (2009) Cochlear implant surgery in patients more than seventy-nine years old. *Laryngoscope* **119**(6):1180–3.
6. Eshraghi AA, Yang NW, Balkany TJ. Comparative study of cochlear damage with three perimodiolar electrode designs. *Laryngoscope.* 2003;**113**(3):415–419. doi:10.1097/00005537-200303000-00005
7. Dhanasingh A, Jolly C. (2017) An overview of cochlear implant electrode array designs. *Hear Res* **356**:93–103.
8. Vaerenberg B, Smits C, De Ceulaer G, *et al.* (2014) Cochlear implant programming: A global survey on the state of the art. *Sci World J* **2014**:501738.
9. Holder JT, Gifford RH. (2021) Effect of increased daily cochlear implant use on auditory perception in adults. *J Speech Lang Hear Res* **64**(10):4044–55.
10. Balkany TJ, Connell SS, Hodges AV, *et al.* (2006) Conservation of residual acoustic hearing after cochlear implantation. *Otol Neurotol* **27**(8):1083–8.
11. Eshraghi AA, Ahmed J, Krysiak E, *et al.* (2017) Clinical, surgical, and electrical factors impacting residual hearing in cochlear implant surgery. *Acta Otolaryngol* **137**(4):384–8.
12. Holder JT, Reynolds SM, Sunderhaus LW, Gifford RH. (2018) Current profile of adults presenting for preoperative cochlear implant evaluation. *Trends Hear* **22**:2331216518755288.
13. Adunka OF, Pillsbury HC, Buchman CA. (2010) Minimizing intracochlear trauma during cochlear implantation. In: Van de Heyning P, Kleine Punte A, eds. *Cochlear Implants and Hearing Preservation*. Basel: Karger Publishers; **67**, 96–107 p. p.
14. Eshraghi AA, Roell J, Shaikh N, *et al.* (2016) A novel combination of drug therapy to protect residual hearing post cochlear implant surgery. *Acta Otolaryngol* **136**(4):420–4.
15. Eshraghi AA, Adil E, He J, *et al.* (2007) Local dexamethasone therapy conserves hearing in an animal model of electrode insertion trauma-induced hearing loss. *Otol Neurotol* **28**(6):842–9.
16. Eshraghi AA, Dinh CT, Bohorquez J, *et al.* (2011) Local drug delivery to conserve hearing: Mechanisms of action of eluted dexamethasone within the cochlea. *Cochlear Implant Int* **12**(suppl 1):S51–3.

17. Hoskison E, Mitchell S, Coulson C. (2017) Systematic review: Radiological and histological evidence of cochlear implant insertion trauma in adult patients. *Cochlear Implants Int* **18**(4):192–7.
18. Santa Maria PL, Domville-Lewis C, Sucher CM, *et al.* (2013) Hearing preservation surgery for cochlear implantation — Hearing and quality of life after 2 years. *Otol Neurotol* **34**(3):526–31.
19. Thomas J, Klein H, Dazert S, Völter C. (2022) Length measurement of cochlear parameters prior to cochlear implantation — Comparison of CT- vs. MRI-based results. *Laryngo-Rhino-Otologie* **101**. doi:10.1055/s-0042-1746813
20. Vazzana C, Stöver T, Helbig S. (2022) Prediction accuracy of cochlear implant electrode insertion depth using a software program. *Laryngo-Rhino-Otologie* **101**. doi:10.1055/s-0042-1746820
21. Müller-Graff FT, Voelker J, Kurz A, *et al.* (2023) Accuracy of radiological prediction of electrode position with otological planning software and implications of high-resolution imaging. *Cochlear Implants Int* **24**(3):144–54.
22. Eshraghi AA, Gupta C, Van De Water TR, *et al.* (2013) Molecular mechanisms involved in cochlear implantation trauma and the protection of hearing and auditory sensory cells by inhibition of c-Jun-N-terminal kinase signaling. *Laryngoscope* **123**(suppl 1):S1–14.
23. Panara K, Shahal D, Mittal R, Eshraghi AA. (2021) Robotics for cochlear implantation surgery: Challenges and opportunities. *Otol Neurotol* **42**(7): e825–35.
24. Caversaccio M, Mantokoudis G, Wagner F, *et al.* (2022) Robotic cochlear implantation for direct cochlear access. *J Vis Exp* (184). doi:10.3791/64047
25. Dombrowski T, Rankovic V, Moser T. (2019) Toward the optical cochlear implant. *Cold Spring Harb Perspect Med* **9**(8):a033225.
26. Rauterkus G, Maxwell AK, Kahane JB, *et al.* (2022) Conversations in cochlear implantation: The inner ear therapy of today. *Biomolecules* **12**(5):649.

11 Management of Single-Sided Deafness

John J. Sheets, AuD[1]; Hillary A. Snapp, PhD, AuD[1]

Abstract

Single-sided deafness (SSD) disrupts spatial hearing, thereby leading to a number of adverse effects for the listener. The functional losses associated with SSD includes reduced sound awareness in the impaired ear, poor speech understanding in noisy environments, and the inability to locate where sound is coming from. These negative consequences are linked to social-emotional impacts, and can result in increased listening effort and overall poorer quality of life in SSD listeners. Clinical rehabilitation of SSD remains limited in its ability to fully restore access to binaural cues to restore spatial hearing abilities. Management of SSD most often consists of rehabilitation through hearing devices and implants, which improves access to sound thus alleviating some of the hearing deficits.

Introduction

Single-sided deafness (SSD) is a condition of complete loss of hearing in one ear with normal or near-normal hearing in the contralateral ear. While there is increasing awareness of the functional deficits associated with bilateral hearing loss, the negative effects of unilateral hearing loss are far less recognized. SSD is characterized by a range of negative functional and psychosocial outcomes.[1] The functional impacts of SSD include inability to

---

Corresponding Author: Hillary A. Snapp, PhD, AuD

[1] Department of Otolaryngology, University of Miami Ear Institute, University of Miami Miller School of Medicine, Miami, FL, United States.

communicate in noisy environments and poor localization abilities, while the reduced sound awareness due to SSD leads to greater uncertainty and requires increased effort to communicate in challenging environments.[2] The psychosocial impacts of this include social withdrawal, activity reduction, increased stress, and feelings of embarrassment.[3] Research suggests that disability and handicap in SSD listeners can meet or exceed that of bilateral hearing loss in some listeners, despite retaining normal hearing in at least one ear.[4]

The etiology and pathogenesis of SSD is broad ranging and the onset of SSD can occur at any point throughout the lifespan. Congenital/early-onset SSD is most commonly due to cochlear nerve deficiency, cytomegalovirus, and inner ear abnormalities, among others.[5] The majority of SSD, however, is acquired and sudden in onset. In these cases, the etiology may be less clear, with over 50% experiencing idiopathic sudden sensorineural hearing loss.[5] When a specific cause can be identified, the most common etiologies for SSD in adults include tumors of cranial nerve VIII, head trauma, chronic otitis media, viral infection, Meniere's disease, and cholesteatoma.[5] Importantly, new or progressive onset of unilateral hearing loss can be the sign of an underlying medical condition and should undergo audiological and medical evaluation as soon as possible. In most cases of SSD, where the unilateral hearing loss is severe to profound, there is little chance for restoration of hearing through drug therapies or surgical intervention.[6] If identified and treated early, some cases of SSD can be improved with steroid treatment although the success of this decreases with time and increasing severity of the loss.[6] When medical treatment is not possible or ineffective, successful management of SSD is possible through the provision of hearing devices and implants.

This chapter will review how hearing with only one ear impacts individuals functionally and what treatment options are available for SSD.

Hearing with Two Ears

It is well established that binaural hearing has many advantages for listeners. Sounds are Characterized by frequency, intensity, and time. In binaural hearing, discrete differences in the timing and loudness of signals between the two ears are processed along the central auditory pathways and integrated in the auditory cortex allowing for enhanced signal-to-noise ratio, detection of sounds, discrimination of sounds, localization of sound sources, and speech intelligibility. These differences are frequency and location dependent, with lower frequency signals providing information about timing and high-frequency signals providing information about signal level. Differences in arrival time at the two ears increases as the signal moves away from mid-line, while the head and torso create an acoustic barrier attenuating signals at the far ear compared to the ear closer to the source. The normal auditory system is highly tuned to these interaural cues, extracting and analyzing minute differences with imperceptible effort.

Listening in Noise

In complex listening environments with multiple talkers or competing environmental noise, processing of auditory cues enables listeners to separate signals of interest (e.g., talkers) from competing signals. This auditory phenomenon becomes increasingly difficult for listeners as the signal-to-noise ratio becomes poorer. Speech intelligibility is particularly affected when the target and the competing signal are co-located. When the target is spatially separated from noise, however, speech intelligibility significantly improves due to the interaural level differences arising from the acoustic head shadow enabling a better signal-to-noise ratio at the ear closer to the target. Here, the head and torso create a physical barrier to the noise interfering with the target signal. This combined with binaural unmasking,[7] where the central auditory system uses the interaural phase and timing differences between the two ears to suppress interfering signals, further contributes to an improved signal-to-noise ratio. In binaural hearing benefits also include the summating of signals at the two ears, increasing the overall perceptual loudness. Collectively, these aspects of binaural hearing contribute to improve listener speech intelligibility in noisy environments.

Localization

Localization of a sound source in space relies on integration of binaural hearing cues and monaural spectral cues in the brainstem and auditory cortex. These cues are frequency dependent, providing different information about where a sound is located in space. Binaural hearing primarily contributes to localization of sounds in the horizontal dimension. Primary cues consist of the interaural timing difference cue primarily salient in the low frequencies below 1,500 Hz; and the interaural level difference cue which increases with frequency.[8] Spectral cues are monaural cues primarily consisting of content above 5,000 Hz. The pinna, head, and torso provide filtering of signals to inform on the direction of the source and contribute to localization in the vertical dimension. Monaural pinna cues can additionally be used to aide localization in the horizontal plane in order to distinguish if a sound originates from the front or rear.[8]

The Monaural Hearing Condition

Single-sided deafness listeners lose access to the important binaural hearing cues that contribute to spatial hearing and speech perception abilities. Individuals with SSD rely on monaural hearing, where only a single ear provides input to the brain, losing access to the critical timing and level difference cues from the two ears.[1] This leads to marked functional impairments in sound source localization and hearing in noise ability for SSD listeners. Factors such as reduced safety that come with poor auditory localization are important considerations in this population.[1] SSD listeners are particularly disadvantaged for sounds arriving at the impaired side due to the acoustic shadowing of the head.[1] In such listening scenarios, low-frequency sounds have long wavelengths enabling them to be well detected at the hearing ear, whereas high-frequency sounds have short wavelengths and are thereby diffracted by head, rendering them imperceptible at the hearing ear. Loss of access to high-frequency cues also negatively effects speech perception, which is compounded in the presence of competing noise in the environment.[1] As a result, a significantly higher signal-to-noise ratio is required at the impaired side relative to the hearing side for SSD listeners to effectively communicate in noisy environments. This impacts not only psychosocial functioning but also performance at school and work.[3] Individuals with SSD often have to employ compensatory strategies, such as turning their head to better exposure of their better hearing ear or positioning communication partners on their better hearing side, to improve the signal-to-noise ratio. This constant adjusting in different situations can lead to increased effort, resulting in greater fatigue in these individuals.[2]

In addition to hearing problems, some patients with SSD may also report tinnitus (ringing/static sound in their ear) or vertigo.[4,5] Bothersome tinnitus may be managed in conjunction with their hearing loss, such as tinnitus counselling. Vertigo should also be evaluated and managed in the otology clinic with vestibular evaluation and consideration of vestibular rehabilitation therapy (VRT) or other medical intervention.

Treatment Options

In the acute stage, SSD may be managed medically through etiology-dependent interventions, such as surgery or steroid injections.[6] For individuals where the hearing loss cannot be remedied through medical intervention, several rehabilitative options exist. These include consideration of a monaural hearing aid for the poorer hearing ear, rerouting the acoustic signal from the poorer hearing side to the better hearing side, and stimulation of the poorer hearing ear with a cochlear implant (CI).[1] Each of these options will be described further.

Use of Hearing Aids in SSD

Traditional hearing aids are utilized to apply amplification of environmental sounds with prescriptive targets for soft, moderate, and loud sounds across the frequency range. This allows for improved perception of sounds for those with mild-to-moderate hearing loss. In individuals with severe-to-profound sensorineural hearing loss, damage to the cochlear and/or neural structures may not allow for effective transmission of auditory signals to the brain. In such cases, residual hearing in the impaired ear may not be enough for the patient to obtain benefit even with use of an appropriate fit hearing aid. Speech perception remains poor and listeners often report the resulting amplified sound to be distorted and intolerable. Individuals with SSD typically have limited-to-no residual hearing in the impaired ear. However, a trial with amplification is encouraged in those with sufficient residual hearing in the impaired ear. Audiological evaluation can help guide recommendation or identify if a monaural hearing aid could be beneficial. Listeners with poor word recognition ability in the impaired ear may perceive reduced benefit, or even interference, with the use traditional hearing aids, which could be evaluated with the use of aided speech perception testing or subjective questionnaires.

Rerouting of Signal

In SSD where the impaired ear cannot be effectively stimulated for hearing rehabilitation, rerouting of signals from the poorer ear side to the better ear can be used to provide listeners with increased access to sound. Rerouting options do not restore access to binaural hearing cues but allow for increased sound awareness and improve the signal-to-noise ratio at the impaired side.[9] While localization and other binaural hearing benefits are not improved, SSD listeners can benefit from reducing the impact of the acoustic head shadow to improve hearing in noise. Primary benefit from rerouting is achieved when the signal of interest and the noise are spatially separated with the target at the impaired ear side. Benefits of rerouting are more limited in diffuse noise settings.

Contralateral routing of signal hearing aid

The traditional form of rerouting of signal is with contralateral routing of signal (CROS) hearing aids. The CROS hearing aid system consists of a microphone and transmitter placed on the deafened ear, which wirelessly sends the signal to a hearing aid worn on the better hearing ear delivered via a receiver in the ear canal. CROS hearing aid systems are advantageous, as if the listener has or acquires hearing loss in the better ear (e.g., due to ageing), amplification can also be applied through the hearing aid in addition to the rerouted signal from the deafened ear.

A primary drawback of CROS devices is the required use of two devices. The reliance of a hearing device in the normal ear can lead to occlusion, even in "open fit" devices.[9] This is of particular importance in children or those with small ear canals. Even when non-occluding, the presence of the hearing aid changes the acoustics of the ear canal, which may interfere with monaural pinna cues.[10] This may further increase the handicap in SSD listeners who are left to solely rely on monaural cues.

Bone conduction device

Rerouting of acoustic signals from the deafened ear to the better hearing ear can also be achieved using bone conduction. Bone conduction devices (BCDs) rely on the bones of the skull to transmit signals transcranially from the impaired side to the better hearing ear. The hearing organ, known as the cochlea, is housed in the temporal bone and its sensory structures are stimulated by sound vibrations, making bone conduction an efficient and effective stimulus pathway.[1] In the case of adults, BCDs are most commonly implanted via a titanium implant placed in the temporal bone which osseointegrates with the temporal bone. Modern surgical options can be percutaneous, with a skin-penetrating abutment, upon which the processor is placed, or active transcutaneous, with a surgically placed implant underneath the skin and external processor attached via magnet. These implantable BCD solutions allow the implant to directly drive the signal, allowing for optimal bone conduction stimulation. BCD device can be applied non-surgically, with use of an adhesive or headband. Non-surgical devices are passive transcutaneous, meaning that the sound must travel across the skin before vibrating the skull. This leads to a frequency-dependent reduction in output of the signal, with the greatest effect occurring in the high frequencies.[11]

Use of a BCD for SSD relies on good hearing in the better hearing ear. The Food and Drug Administration (FDA) allows for use of BCD devices in SSD patients with normal hearing (20 dB HL or better) in the better hearing ear.[12] This is due to the limited output of BCDs, and attenuation that may occur with the sound transmission across the skull. As a consideration, patients pursuing BCD for SSD must be counselled that benefit from the device may be reduced in the future if hearing loss in the better hearing ear develops.

One benefit of rerouting with a BCD is the allowance of the normal hearing ear to remain completely open, not obstructing the ear canal with use of a device only on the deaf-ear side.[1] The primary drawback of BCDs is the more invasive nature of an implant, particularly for individuals who may have skin healing difficulties or are unable to undergo general anesthesia. Although of low incidence, percutaneous BCDs have a skin-penetrating abutment, which may lead to skin complications.[13] Active transcutaneous devices require use of an implanted magnet, which in some cases limits the use of magnetic resonance imaging (MRI) without removal of the internal magnet. In other cases, imaging may be impacted by artefact from the magnet. This can be of high importance for individuals with a history of head tumors, such as vestibular schwannoma. Additionally, BCD should not be considered as a primary option for individuals with asymmetric hearing loss, per the guidelines set by the FDA.[12]

Cochlear Implant

A CI is the only available solution that can be used to provide direct stimulation to the deafened ear. CIs use electrical contacts inside the cochlea to provide direct electrical stimulation to the auditory nerve. This is done through the surgical implantation of an electrode array into the cochlea and use of an external sound processor. CIs have long been used in individuals with bilateral moderate-to-profound sensorineural hearing loss who do not benefit from use of traditional hearing aids. Direct electrical stimulation of the deaf ear with a CI in combination with the better hearing ear allows for some binaural input to the brain. As such CIs provide specific hearing benefits to SSD listeners over rerouting such as improved localization performance and speech understanding in the deaf ear.[14] Despite this, performance with CI for SSD has been shown to be variable between individuals and, overall, continues to lag that of individuals with normal hearing.[1] This is mostly attributed to the limited ability of a CI to provide reliable hearing cues for binaural hearing restoration.[1] CIs provide a listener with loudness cues that can be reliably used to facilitate location of a sound source, but do not provide reliable interaural timing difference cues. An additional benefit of the use of CIs in SSD listeners is the reduced perception of tinnitus with the use of a CI, with one study showing improved or completely resolved tinnitus perception in 81% of patients.[14]

In traditional CI candidates, a number of variables have been shown to impact speech performance outcomes, such as etiology, duration of hearing loss, use of hearing aids prior to implantation and age.[15] Although similar variables should be considered with SSD, special considerations should be made particularly for those undergoing CI for SSD. The etiology of hearing loss is a primary component when considering CI for SSD. For example, cochlear nerve deficiency has been shown to be present in as much as 50% of children with SSD,[5] which would likely result in sub-optimal outcomes with a CI and, ultimately, device rejection.[16] Cytomegalovirus, another primary etiology for SSD in children, can be concomitant with significant neurocognitive deficits.[17] For this reason, families considering CI for SSD in children with cytomegalovirus should be heavily counselled on possible limited benefit from CI, given central nervous system deficits. Duration of deafness has been shown to be correlated with outcomes in bilateral CI recipients; however, there is limited evidence to estimate the relationship of duration of deafness and CI in SSD listeners.[18]

While CI for SSD may be useful for some individuals, additional consideration should be given to such etiologies where performance is likely to be poor or limited benefit is anticipated such as vestibular schwannoma, auditory neuropathy, or cochlear malformation. Regardless of etiology or other patient factors, clear and transparent counselling, including possible positive or negative outcomes, must be offered prior to moving forward with cochlear implantation for individuals with SSD, given the large variability in outcomes.

Conclusion

Single-sided deafness leads to significant functional and quality of life impacts in many individuals. Hearing with one ear results in increased difficulty listening in noise, challenges telling where sounds are coming from, and increased listening effort in daily listening situations. Medical assessment and treatment are vital in the acute phase of sudden-onset SSD, but several audiological treatment options are available for those with permanent SSD, including CROS hearing aids, bone conduction devices and cochlear implantation. CROS hearing aids offer a non-surgical option to relieve some of the deficits that come with SSD, while BCDs allow for this access with the use of only one device. CIs have become a much more common treatment tool for SSD, but outcomes and restoration of binaural hearing continues to be explored. Regardless of the treatment option pursued, patient motivation and appropriate counselling are key to positive outcomes in these individuals.

References

1. Snapp HA, Ausili SA. (2020) Hearing with one ear: Consequences and treatments for profound unilateral hearing loss. *J Clin Med* **9**(4):1010.
2. Alhanbali S, Dawes P, Lloyd S, Munro KJ. Self-reported listening-related effort and fatigue in hearing-impaired adults. *Ear Hear* **38**(1):e39–48.
3. Lucas L, Katiri R, Kitterick PT. (2018) The psychological and social consequences of single-sided deafness in adulthood. *Int J Audiol* **57**(1):21–30.
4. Sano H, Okamoto M, Ohhashi K, *et al.* (2013) Quality of life reported by patients with idiopathic sudden sensorineural hearing loss. *Otol Neurotol* **34**(1):36–40.
5. Usami SI, Kitoh R, Moteki H, *et al.* (2017) Etiology of single-sided deafness and asymmetrical hearing loss. *Acta Otolaryngol* **137**(sup565):S2–7.
6. Haynes DS, O'Malley M, Cohen S, *et al.* (2007) Intratympanic dexamethasone for sudden sensorineural hearing loss after failure of systemic therapy. *Laryngoscope* **117**(1):3–15.
7. Durlach NI. (1963) Equalization and cancellation theory of binaural masking-level differences. *J Acoust Soc Am* **35**(8):1206–18.
8. Blauert J. (1996) *Spatial Hearing: The Psychophysics of Human Sound Localisation.* Harvard, MA: The MIT Press.
9. Snapp H. (2019) Nonsurgical management of single-sided deafness: Contralateral routing of signal. *J Neurol Surg B Skull Base* **80**(2):132–8.
10. Pedley AJ, Kitterick PT. (2017) Contralateral routing of signals disrupts monaural level and spectral cues to sound localisation on the horizontal plane. *Hear Res* **353**:104–11.
11. Beros S, Dobrev I, Farahmandi TS, *et al.* (2022) Transcutaneous and percutaneous bone conduction sound propagation in single-sided deaf patients and cadaveric heads. *Int J Audiol* **61**(8):678–85.
12. Food and Drug Administation Center for Devices and Radiological Health. (2021) *Approval Letter for Cochlear Baha 6 System.*
13. Gluth MB, Eager KM, Eikelboom RH, Atlas MD. (2010) Long-term benefit perception, complications, and device malfunction rate of bone-anchored hearing aid implantation for profound unilateral sensorineural hearing loss. *Otol Neurotol* **31**(9):1427–34.
14. Deep NL, Spitzer ER, Shapiro WH, *et al.* (2021) Cochlear implantation in adults with single-sided deafness: Outcomes and device use. *Otol Neurotol* **42**(3):414–23.
15. Smulders YE, Hendriks T, Eikelboom RH, *et al.* (2017) Predicting sequential cochlear implantation performance: A systematic review. *Audiol Neurootol* **22**(6):356–63.

16. Buchman CA, Teagle HF, Roush PA, *et al.* (2011) Cochlear implantation in children with labyrinthine anomalies and cochlear nerve deficiency: Implications for auditory brainstem implantation. *Laryngoscope* **121**(9):1979–88.
17. Kraaijenga VJC, Van Houwelingen F, Van der Horst SF, *et al.* (2018) Cochlear implant performance in children deafened by congenital cytomegalovirus — a systematic review. *Clin Otolaryngol* **43**(5):1283–95.
18. Kurz A, Grubenbecher M, Rak K, *et al.* (2019) The impact of etiology and duration of deafness on speech perception outcomes in SSD patients. *Eur Arch Otorhinolaryngol* **276**(12):3317–25.

12 Recent Advancements in Developing Drug Therapy for Auditory Disorders

Alexa Denton, MD[1,2]*; Dimitri A. Godur, BS[1]*; Jaimee N. Cooper, BS[1]; Jeenu Mittal, MSc[1]; Adamya Aggarwal, BS[1]; Keelin McKenna, BS[1,2]; Soumil Prasad, BS[1]; Devin J. Kennedy, BS[1]; Moeed Moosa, BS[1]; Adrien A Eshraghi, MD, MSc, FACS[1]; Rahul Mittal, PhD[1]

Abstract

Medical management of auditory disorders has proved to be a challenging area of study. Due to the various underlying causes of these disorders, individuals have a wide spectrum of symptoms, from temporary to permanent changes in hearing. In addition to this disparity in physical presentation, there are challenges in developing medications, such as understanding the clinical course of a patient's symptoms as well as the difficulties in targeting the inner ear due to the presence of the blood labyrinth barrier, a barrier between the blood vessels and the inner ear. This chapter aims to review some of the recent advancements in developing treatment modalities for the medical management of auditory disorders such as sudden sensorineural hearing loss, idiopathic sensorineural hearing loss, noise-induced hearing loss, cispla-

---

Corresponding Author: Rahul Mittal, PhD

Hearing Research and Cochlear Implant Laboratory, Department of Otolaryngology, University of Miami Miller School of Medicine, 1600 NW 10th Avenue, Miami, FL, United States.

*These authors have contributed equally to this work

[1] Hearing Research and Cochlear Implant Laboratory, Department of Otolaryngology, University of Miami Miller School of Medicine, Miami, FL, United States.

[2] Herbert Wertheim College of Medicine, Florida International University, Miami, FL, United States.

tin ototoxicity, antibiotic ototoxicity, tinnitus, vertigo, and Meniere's disease. Corticosteroids have been used extensively to alleviate symptoms in individuals with hearing loss and vestibular problems. Various medical combinations have been compared to and used in conjunction with corticosteroids with varied outcomes. Antioxidants also play a role in treating many conditions. The efficacy and safety of other off-label and novel medications were evaluated in preliminary studies based on animal models. The efficacy and safety of other off-label and novel medications were evaluated in preliminary studies based on animal models; results were varied. Future research should continue looking for novel drug candidates for the efficient treatment of auditory disorders due to the discrepancy in outcomes and incomplete understanding of the mechanisms of action of both disorders and treatments.

Keywords: auditory disorders, medical management, hearing loss, tinnitus, vertigo, Meniere's disease

Introduction

Auditory disorders mainly include isolated or combinations of symptoms such as hearing loss, tinnitus, and vertigo.[1] While there have been advancements in outlining the pathophysiology of some of these conditions (idiopathic SNHL), the lack of complete understanding has led to difficulties in developing feasible treatment modalities for patients.[1] In addition to the challenges in developing medications, the blood-labyrinth barrier, the barrier between the fluid in the inner ear and the blood vessels of the inner ear, prevents most compounds from accessing the inner ear.[2] This has prompted the exploration of oral drugs along with treatments locally delivered into the inner ear.[1]

The inner ear conditions that will be discussed throughout this chapter include sudden sensorineural hearing loss (SSNHL), idiopathic sensorineural hearing loss (SNHL), noise-induced hearing loss (NIHL), cisplatin ototoxicity, antibiotic ototoxicity, tinnitus, vertigo, and Meniere's disease. Although medicinal, surgical, and behavioral treatments have been used in research trials to reduce the impact of these specific illnesses and accompanying symptoms, no medications are currently FDA-approved for clinicians to provide to patients for sensorineural hearing loss.[1]

Auditory Disorders and Their Medical Management

Hearing Loss

Sudden sensorineural hearing loss

A common early treatment for SSNHL is systemic oral corticosteroids (Table 12.1). One interesting trial looked at the efficacy of pulse steroid treatment for SSNHL. One treatment group received 500mg IV methylprednisolone

Table 12.1 Medications studied to treat hearing loss in clinical trials.

Medication	Condition	Drug class	Proposed mechanism of action	References
Prednisolone, prednisone	Sudden sensorineural hearing loss (SSNHL), idiopathic SNHL; noise induced hearing loss (NIHL)	Corticosteroid	Decrease inflammation	Eftekharian *et al.*,[3] Marx *et al.*,[4] Mirian *et al.*[5]
Insulin-like growth factor (IGF-1)	SSNHL	Peptide hormone	Hair cell protection	Marx *et al.*[4]
Heparin	Idiopathic SNHL	Anticoagulant	Minimizes inflammation, anticoagulation	Kim *et al.*[6]
Ebselen	NIHL	Seleno-organic molecule	Mimics glutathione peroxidase, prevents loss of inner hair cell damage, antioxidant	Kil *et al.*[7]
Kenpaullone, magnesium-aspartate, carbogen, vitamin C and B12, and alpha-lipoic acid	NIHL	Antioxidants	Prevent reactive oxygen species (ROS) damage	Teitz *et al.*[8], Gupta *et al.*[9]
Sodium thiosulfate	Cisplatin-induced hearing loss (CIHL)	Antioxidant	Prevents ROS damage	Freyer *et al.*[10]
Vitamin E	Cisplatin ototoxicity	Antioxidant	Prevent ROS damage	Villani *et al.*[12]

(*Continued*)

Table 12.1 (*Continued*)

Medication	Condition	Drug class	Proposed mechanism of action	References
Atorvastatin	Cisplatin ototoxicity	HMG-CoA reductase inhibitor (cholesterol medication)	Anti-oxidative stress properties, decreased inflammation, improved microcirculation	Fernandez *et al.*, 2020.[11]
N-acetylcysteine (NAC)	Antibiotic ototoxicity	Antioxidant	Prevents ROS damage, anti-oxidant	Vural *et al.*[13]

for three consecutive days, followed by 1mg/kg of oral prednisolone for 11 days. The other group received 1mg/kg of oral prednisolone for 14 days. They found that the pulse steroids (500mg IV methylprednisolone) was no more effective than a traditional 14-day course of prednisolone.[3]

Corticosteroid pulse treatment (3 days of high dose steroid followed by 11 days of traditional dosing) with prednisolone has not demonstrated any clear advantages over typical tapering oral medication; however, both groups had limited sample numbers and require additional investigation.[3] The use of insulin-like growth factor-1 (IGF-1), a hormone that promotes tissue development, is currently being investigated in small pilot studies as a potential treatment modality for SSNHL. This topical IGF-1 treatment can preserve inner ear hair cells that have been damaged to varying degrees.[4] Logically, the longer a patient has SSNHL, the less effective IGF-1 treatment is. Furthermore, trials utilizing trans-tympanic topical IGF-1 treatment show recovery in slightly more than 50% with patients reporting side effects of pain, dizziness, and headache.[4]

Idiopathic sensorineural hearing loss

Treatments and pharmacological choices for idiopathic SNHL (hearing loss caused by unknown factors) are comparable to those for non-idiopathic SNHL, with the most frequent being a tapering course of oral corticosteroids like prednisone.[5] Combinations of other well-known medications have also demonstrated potential benefits in idiopathic cases. For instance, heparin, an anticoagulant, is not recommended on its own because of its potential side effects, yet it has been shown to be beneficial in combination with corticosteroids to improve hearing. This is perhaps due to its involvement in reducing inner ear inflammation and improving blood flow; nonetheless, further research is needed to determine its efficacy.[6]

Noise-induced hearing loss

There are many drugs that are currently being investigated to target NIHL, such as antioxidants that prevent damage from harmful substances causing oxidative stress.[7] One such compound with promising results is ebselen, a small molecule that mimics the enzyme glutathione peroxidase 1 (GPx1), which neutralizes oxidative damage caused by acoustic trauma.[7] Other antioxidant substances have been tried and are shown to have positive effects. Some of these include kenpaullone [a cyclin-dependent kinase 2 (CDK2) inhibitor], Mg-aspartate, N-acetylcysteine (NAC), carbogen, vitamins C and B12, and alpha-lipoic acid (ALA); however, further studies and clinical trials are needed to determine the efficacy these medications for NIHL.[8,9]

Ototoxicity

Cisplatin-induced ototoxicity

A majority of the medications studied in preventing and/or treating cisplatin-induced hearing loss have been used due to their antioxidant effect (Table 12.1).[10,11] Sodium thiosulfate, a sodium-containing antioxidant, directly neutralizes cisplatin and ultimately protects from the toxic products of cisplatin which damage the inner ear. It has been the most widely studied medication to prevent cisplatin-induced ototoxicity.[10] Although this medication can decrease the risk of ototoxicity, it can also potentially affect the therapeutic levels needed for cisplatin to treat cancer. Studies have evaluated intravenous administration of sodium thiosulfate and its effect on reducing ototoxicity.[10] It has been proposed that sodium thiosulfate might be utilized to prevent cisplatin-induced hearing loss without reducing cisplatin's anti-cancer activity, when used locally (intratympanic injection). There are currently clinical trials ongoing evaluating its efficacy with local administration.[10]

Vitamin E and atorvastatin are two other medications that have been investigated as treatment modalities for cisplatin induced hearing loss.[11] Vitamin E, a well-known antioxidant, was given daily to patients in a small study with successful results. The treatment group, receiving Vitamin E (400mg per day) was found to have improved hearing at 2000Hz and 8000Hz when compared to a control group.[12] Furthermore, atorvastatin, a cholesterol-lowering medicine, has been demonstrated to offer anti-oxidative stress effects as well as protection against hearing loss in individuals with head and neck cancer, indicating the need for further studies with larger sample size.[11]

Antibiotic ototoxicity

In addition to cisplatin toxicity, many clinical trials have investigated antioxidants to protect against damage from antibiotics such as aminoglycosides. In a study by Vural et al., patients with end stage renal disease who had received amikacin, a known ototoxic antibiotic, were randomized to receive either 600mg of NAC orally two times a day and peritoneal dialysis (PD) or PD alone. All participants received audiometry prior to treatment, one month, and one year after treatment. They found that the group who received NAC had a trend towards better pure tone averages (PTAs) compared to the control, but this data did not reach statistical significance. NAC is currently being investigated as a treatment for various hearing disorders.

Tinnitus and Vestibular Conditions

Tinnitus

Many well-known drugs used to treat other conditions have also been used to treat tinnitus symptoms in patients. While the FDA has not reached a definitive decision regarding approval of medications for patients experiencing tinnitus symptoms, some useful classes of medications include corticosteroids, nerve blockers, fluoxetine, anti-anxiety medicines, and anti-depressants.[14–17] An interesting study determined the efficacy of the anti-inflammatory effects of an injection of dexamethasone into the inner ear and produced positive results.[14] Furthermore, nerve blockers such as lidocaine have long been prescribed as a therapeutic tool. Due to the risks of using intravenous lidocaine, the use of trans-dermal lidocaine patches has been evaluated.[15] Participants' tinnitus intensity improved after 1 month of therapy with lidocaine patches, although several patients discontinued participating and affected the power of the study.[15]

Anti-anxiety and anti-depressant medications have been used in patients with tinnitus, both to combat the psychiatric effects that tinnitus causes and the influence they have on the ringing sensation itself. A recent study explored the usage of the anti-depressant and anti-anxiety drug fluoxetine alone or in combination with the anti-anxiety drug alprazolam, a benzodiazepine.[16] Both medications have been used alone to treat tinnitus, with varying degrees of success. This study discovered that both treatment groups saw a trend towards a reduction in tinnitus severity, with no statistically significant difference in improvement, indicating that combination therapy might be explored in future research. Acamprosate, which is typically used to treat alcohol dependency, has also been studied to reduce tinnitus.[17] Acamprosate effectively alleviated tinnitus symptoms despite participant variability in research with a limited sample size and a short-term follow-up of 30 days.[17]

Vertigo

Various therapy techniques, including exercises and nutritional adjustments, have been utilized to clinically ameliorate symptoms depending on the diagnostic category of vertigo (Table 12.2). Scoltz *et al.* compared the antihistamine betahistine alone and an antihistamine combination drug containing cinnarizine and dimenhydrinate. They discovered that individuals with peripheral vestibular vertigo who were given cinnarizine and dimenhydrinate had more substantial decreases in vertigo symptoms than those who just received betahistine.[18] These trials show the potential use of antihypertensives and antihistamines as a combination treatment for individuals suffering from vertigo due to peripheral vestibular vertigo.

Methylprednisolone, a corticosteroid, may also help with vertigo symptoms. Patients who received methylprednisolone had a reduced need for repositioning therapy, suggesting that the benefits of corticosteroids may be investigated for treatment of persistent BPPV.[19] Patients who received methylprednisolone had a reduced need for repositioning therapy, suggesting that corticosteroids should be investigated for treatment of persistent BPPV.[19]

Beta blockers, a commonly used class of anti-hypertensives, has been studied as a prophylactic medication for individuals with vestibular migraine. In a clinical trial by Salviz *et al.*, propranolol, a beta blocker, and

Table 12.2 Medications studied to treat auditory disorders.

Medication	Condition	Drug class	Proposed mechanism of action	References
Dexamethasone	Tinnitus, Meniere's disease	Corticosteroid	Decreases inflammation	Yener *et al.*,[14] Lambert *et al.*,[21] Albu *et al.*[22]
Lidocaine	Tinnitus	Anesthetic	Nerve blocker that leads to control of brain hyperactivity	O'Brien *et al.*[15]
Acamprosate	Tinnitus	γ-Aminobutyric acid (GABA) agonist and glutamate antagonist	Inhibits brain hyperactivity	Farhadi *et al.*[17]
Fluoxetine ± alprazolam	Tinnitus	Selective serotonin reuptake inhibitor (SSRI) ± benzodiazepine	Reduce anxiety associated with tinnitus and unknown mechanism for tinnitus severity	Saberi *et al.*[16]
Cinnarizine	Peripheral vestibular vertigo	Calcium channel blocker (antihypertensive)	Unknown	Scholtz *et al.*[18]
Betahistine	Peripheral vestibular vertigo	Antihistamine (strong antagonist of H3, weak agonist of H1)	Unknown	Scholtz *et al.*,[18] Albu *et al.*[22]
Methylprednisolone	Vestibular neuritis, benign paroxysmal positional vertigo (BPPV); Meniere's disease	Corticosteroid	Reduces inflammation	Pérez *et al.*[19]
Propranolol	Vestibular migraine	Beta-blocker (antihypertensive)	Inhibits nervous system hyperactivity	Salviz *et al.*[20]
Venlafaxine	Vestibular migraine	Serotonin norepinephrine reuptake inhibitor (antidepressant)	Anxiolytic	Salviz *et al.*[20]
Gentamicin	Meniere's disease	Aminoglycoside antibiotic	Reduction of type 1 hair cells in all five vestibular organs	Scarpa *et al.*,[23] Sam *et al.*,[24] Patel *et al.*[25]

venlafaxine, an antidepressant, were comparatively studied in a randomized clinical trial. Both venlafaxine and propranolol were shown to be effective in reducing dizziness handicap scores and vertigo severity scores, indicating a reduction in vestibular migraine symptoms. Although, venlafaxine was more effective at alleviating depressive symptoms in this cohort. Further studies are ongoing to understand their efficacy.[20]

Meniere's disease

Recent research has looked at medications and their usage in Meniere's disease, specifically those that target hearing loss, tinnitus, and vertigo symptoms. These include corticosteroids, antibiotics, and antihistamines, which are used to treat a variety of symptoms (Table 12.2). Lambert *et al.* investigated the effects of dexamethasone injections into the middle ear on vertigo, tinnitus, and hearing safety. They discovered that these injections did not have detrimental effects on hearing, improved overall vertigo rates in patients, but had no effect on any tinnitus scales.[21]

Albu *et al.* investigated the addition of oral betahistine to intratympanic dexamethasone injections to assess symptom improvements and discovered that this combination treatment decreased vertigo symptoms but did not improve hearing levels or tinnitus ratings.[22] This may imply that betahistine is beneficial in Meniere's; however, the effect on hearing loss with the addition of a corticosteroid is insufficient at this time and warrants further studies. Similarly, despite the risk of causing hearing loss, low-dose gentamicin administration to the middle ear has been advocated as a medical therapy for vertigo symptoms in Meniere's disease, with promising outcomes in reducing vertigo episodes while avoiding cochlear damage.[23] Sam *et al.* also showed a decrease in vertigo episodes and an improvement in tinnitus symptoms with transtympanic gentamicin; however, they did have participants who reported hearing loss, suggesting the need for further studies to evaluate gentamicin dosage as a therapeutic tool in Meniere's disease.[24] Lastly, Patel *et al.* compared the use of methylprednisolone injections with gentamicin in the treatment of vertigo in Meniere's disease. It was observed that both groups had a decrease in the average frequency of vertigo episodes, but not between groups. Interestingly, patients in the gentamicin group had greater difficulty with speech perception, suggesting the possible side effects of gentamicin on hearing.[25] These studies, which focused on various drugs and particular symptoms, demonstrate the ongoing medical challenges in controlling Menieres disease. Because of the risk of associated hearing loss with intratympanic gentamicin and the fact that Menières disease can be bilateral in many patients, we prefer other treatment modalities. Currently, there is an ongoing clinical trial looking at the efficacy of Ebselen in Menières, but the results are not available at this time.

Conclusions and Future Directions

Clinical studies have resulted in advances in the medical care of inner ear disease, using both known and novel drugs; yet the absence of equivalent outcomes between trials using the same medications continues to make FDA clearance difficult to obtain. This might be attributed to a lack of understanding of disease pathophysiology, the variety of disease manifestations, and the unknown therapeutic mechanism of action in symptomatic relief. For both hearing loss and vestibular disorders, corticosteroids and antioxidants play the most important role in symptom relief, but they may not be sufficient on their own. Other studies have examined several substances in combination and individually, such as some psychiatric medications, such as psychiatric medications; however, the results varied. Due to the wide variety of findings observed in these trials, additional investigations should be conducted in the future to further advise medical therapy and developing novel effective interventions for auditory disorders.

References

1. Nyberg S, Abbott NJ, Shi X, *et al.* (2019) Delivery of therapeutics to the inner ear: The challenge of the blood-labyrinth barrier. *Sci Transl Med* **11**(482):eaao0935. doi:10.1126/scitranslmed.aao0935.
2. Denton AJ, Godur DA, Mittal J, *et al.* (2022) Recent advancements in understanding the gut microbiome and the inner ear axis. *Otolaryngol Clin North Am* **55**(5):1125–37.
3. Eftekharian A, Amizadeh M. (2016) Pulse steroid therapy in idiopathic sudden sensorineural hearing loss: A randomized controlled clinical trial. *Laryngoscope* **126**(1):150–5. doi:10.1002/lary.25244.
4. Marx M, Younes E, Chandrasekhar SS, *et al.* (2018) International consensus (ICON) on treatment of sudden sensorineural hearing loss. *Eur Ann Otorhinolaryngol Head Neck Dis* **135**(1S):S23–8. doi:10.1016/j.anorl.2017.12.011.

5. Mirian C, Ovesen T. (2020) Intratympanic vs systemic corticosteroids in first-line treatment of idiopathic sudden sensorineural hearing loss: A systematic review and meta-analysis. *JAMA Otolaryngol Head Neck Surg* **146**(5):421–8. doi:10.1001/jamaoto.2020.0047.
6. Kim J, Jeong J, Ha R, Sunwoo W. (2020) Heparin therapy as adjuvant treatment for profound idiopathic sudden sensorineural hearing loss. *Laryngoscope* **130**(5):1310–5. doi:10.1002/lary.28231.
7. Kil J, Lobarinas E, Spankovich C, *et al.* (2017) Safety and efficacy of ebselen for the prevention of noise-induced hearing loss: A randomised, double-blind, placebo-controlled, phase 2 trial. *Lancet* **390**(10098):969–79. doi:10.1016/S0140-6736(17)31791-9.
8. Teitz T, Fang J, Goktug AN, *et al.* (2018) CDK2 inhibitors as candidate therapeutics for cisplatin- and noise-induced hearing loss. *J Exp Med* **215**(4):1187–203. doi:10.1084/jem.20172246.
9. Gupta A, Koochakzadeh S, Nguyen SA, *et al.* (2021) Pharmacological prevention of noise-induced hearing loss: A systematic review. *Otol Neurotol* **42**(1):2–9. doi:10.1097/MAO.0000000000002858.
10. Freyer DR, Chen L, Krailo MD, *et al.* (2017) Effects of sodium thiosulfate versus observation on development of cisplatin-induced hearing loss in children with cancer (ACCL0431): A multicentre, randomised, controlled, open-label, phase 3 trial. *Lancet Oncol* **18**(1):63–74. doi:10.1016/S1470-2045(16)30625-8.
11. Fernandez KA, Allen P, Campbell M, *et al.* (2021) Atorvastatin is associated with reduced cisplatin-induced hearing loss. *J Clin Invest* **131**(1):e142616. doi:10.1172/JCI142616.
12. Villani V, Zucchella C, Cristalli G, *et al.* (2016) Vitamin E neuroprotection against cisplatin ototoxicity: Preliminary results from a randomized, placebo-controlled trial. *Head Neck* **38**(Suppl 1):E2118–21. doi:10.1002/hed.24396.
13. Vural A, Koçyiğit İ, Şan F, *et al.* (2018) Long-term protective effect of n-acetylcysteine against amikacin-induced ototoxicity in end-stage renal disease: A randomized trial. *Perit Dial Int* **38**(1):57–62. doi:10.3747/pdi.2017.00133.
14. Yener HM, Sarı E, Aslan M, *et al.* (2020) The efficacy of intratympanic steroid injection in tinnitus cases unresponsive to medical treatment. *J Int Adv Otol* **16**(2):197–200. doi:10.5152/iao.2020.7588.
15. O'Brien DC, Robinson AD, Wang N, Diaz R. (2019) Transdermal lidocaine as treatment for chronic subjective tinnitus: A pilot study. *Am J Otolaryngol* **40**(3):413–7. doi:10.1016/j.amjoto.2019.03.009.
16. Saberi A, Nemati S, Lili EK, *et al.* (2021) Investigating the efficacy of fluoxetine vs. fluoxetine plus alprazolam (single therapy vs. combination therapy) in treatment of chronic tinnitus: A placebo-controlled study. *Am J Otolaryngol* **42**(3):102898. doi:10.1016/j.amjoto.2020.102898.

17. Farhadi M, Salem MM, Asghari A, *et al.* (2020) Impact of acamprosate on chronic tinnitus: A randomized-controlled trial. *Ann Otol Rhinol Laryngol* **129**(11):1110–9. doi:10.1177/0003489420930773.
18. Scholtz AW, Hahn A, Stefflova B, *et al.* (2019) Efficacy and safety of a fixed combination of cinnarizine 20 mg and dimenhydrinate 40 mg vs betahistine dihydrochloride 16 mg in patients with peripheral vestibular vertigo: A prospective, multinational, multicenter, double-blind, randomized, non-inferiority clinical trial. *Clin Drug Investig* **39**(11):1045–56. doi:10.1007/s40261-019-00858-6.
19. Pérez P, Franco V, Oliva M, López Escámez JA. (2016) A pilot study using intratympanic methylprednisolone for treatment of persistent posterior canal benign paroxysmal positional vertigo. *J Int Adv Otol* **12**(3):321–5. doi:10.5152/iao.2016.3014.
20. Salviz M, Yuce T, Acar H, *et al.* (2016) Propranolol and venlafaxine for vestibular migraine prophylaxis: A randomized controlled trial. *Laryngoscope* **126**(1):169–74. doi:10.1002/lary.25445.
21. Lambert PR, Carey J, Mikulec AA, LeBel C; Otonomy Ménière's Study Group. (2016) Intratympanic sustained-exposure dexamethasone thermosensitive gel for symptoms of Ménière's disease: Randomized phase 2b safety and efficacy trial. *Otol Neurotol* **37**(10):1669–76. doi:10.1097/MAO.0000000000001227.
22. Albu S, Nagy A, Doros C, *et al.* (2016) Treatment of Meniere's disease with intratympanic dexamethasone plus high dosage of betahistine. *Am J Otolaryngol* **37**(3):225–30. doi:10.1016/j.amjoto.2015.12.007.
23. Scarpa A, Ralli M, Cassandro C, *et al.* (2019) Low-dose intratympanic gentamicin administration for unilateral Meniere's disease using a method based on clinical symptomatology: Preliminary results. *Am J Otolaryngol* **40**(6):102289. doi:10.1016/j.amjoto.2019.102289.
24. Sam G, Chung DW, van der Hoeven R, *et al.* (2016) The effect of intratympanic gentamicin for treatment of Ménière's disease on lower frequency hearing. *Int J Clin Pharm* **38**(4):780–3. doi:10.1007/s11096-016-0295-4.
25. Patel M, Agarwal K, Arshad Q, *et al.* (2016) Intratympanic methylprednisolone versus gentamicin in patients with unilateral Ménière's disease: A randomised, double-blind, comparative effectiveness trial. *Lancet* **388**(10061):2753–62. doi:10.1016/S0140-6736(16)31461-1.
26. Bayer O, Adrion C, Al Tawil A, *et al.*; PROVEMIG investigators. (2019) Results and lessons learnt from a randomized controlled trial: Prophylactic treatment of vestibular migraine with metoprolol (PROVEMIG). *Trials* **20**(1):813. doi:10.1186/s13063-019-3903-5.

13 Progress and Challenges for Gene Therapy for Hearing and Balance Disorders

Aziz El-Amraoui, PhD[1]

Abstract

Hearing loss is a prevalent condition that affects millions globally. While hearing aids and implants alleviate the burden, personalized hearing medicine and inner ear therapeutics offer promising solutions. Gene therapies (gene replacement and gene editing) have demonstrated effectiveness in animal models, and ongoing studies continue to tackle the remaining challenges for their clinical translation. Maintaining baso-apical cochlear spatial tonotopic organization, selecting optimal vectors according to target cell types, and *routes* of administration for gene delivery, discovering new efficient nuclease variants, and identifying precise clinical endpoints are key considerations. The safety and efficacy of these therapies must be rigorously evaluated, particularly regarding immune responses and the overall safety of surgical procedures and gene delivery vectors. While challenges remain, ongoing research and collaborations between scientists, clinicians, audiologists, engineers, academic, private companies, patient organizations, and regulatory bodies are necessary to overcome obstacles and pave the way for effective and safe personalized inner ear therapies.

Corresponding Author: Aziz El-Amraoui, PhD
Institut Pasteur, Institut de l'Audition, Université Paris Cité, INSERM AO06, Unit Progressive Sensory Disorders, Pathophysiology and Therapy, Paris, France.
[1] Institut Pasteur, Institut de l'Audition, Université Paris Cité, INSERM AO06, Unit Progressive Sensory Disorders, Pathophysiology and Therapy, Paris, France.

Introduction

Hearing loss is the most common sensory deficit, affecting all age groups from children (1 in 500) to the elderly (over 50% of those aged 75 and over) (see http://www.who.int/). Today, hearing loss is the fourth leading cause of disability globally. It can be caused by a variety of factors, including genetic factors, aging, acoustic trauma, ototoxic drugs such as aminoglycosides, and exposure to loud sounds.[1–4]

Currently, there is no curative treatment for sensorineural hearing loss. Rehabilitation methods, such as conventional hearing aids and, for severe cases, cochlear implants, are used to manage hearing loss. Although research aims to improve the performance of prosthetic hearing devices, particularly in restoring better speech perception in noise and satisfactory music perception, new therapeutic approaches are being explored. The design of effective therapies for the inner ear requires comprehensive consideration of the broad spectrum of phenotypic characteristics associated with deafness. Deafness manifests in various ways, influenced by multiple underlying causes and involving different target cells within the auditory system. These crucial factors must be carefully analyzed to develop appropriate treatment strategies. Tailored approaches that address the specific factors contributing to an individual's deafness can lead to more successful outcomes. By gaining a deeper understanding of the intricate complexities of deafness, researchers can devise personalized therapeutic interventions aimed at restoring or enhancing auditory function, thereby improving the quality of life for individuals affected by this condition.

Hearing loss is an extremely heterogeneous disorder, potentially involving up to 1,000 different genes. These genes can directly cause deafness (Mendelian) or amplify the effects of environmental or personal risk factors. Currently, around 140 deafness genes have been identified, but many more are yet to be discovered (see http://hereditaryhearingloss.org/). The growing understanding of molecular mechanisms and the pivotal role of molecules in sensory cells and associated neurons has ushered in a new era of possibilities for personalized gene therapies. Advances in research have shed light on the intricate workings of these cells, unravelling the complex interactions and pathways involved in sensory perception. Capitalizing on this knowledge, scientists now have the opportunity to develop targeted gene therapies that can address specific genetic abnormalities or dysfunctions underlying sensory disorders. By tailoring treatments to an individual's unique genetic makeup, these innovative therapies hold the promise of restoring or enhancing sensory function, providing new avenues of hope for individuals affected by these conditions.[1,3] Gene therapy is currently the subject of over 3,000 ongoing clinical trials, and insights gained from these trials could greatly enhance the design and implementation of gene therapy for cochlear and vestibular disorders.[1,4] In this chapter, we will emphasize the potential of gene therapy as a promising approach to prevent or slow loss of hearing and/or balance. We will closely examine areas that require advancement to expand the application of gene therapy in the clinical treatment of hearing loss. These areas include the identification of safe and effective delivery routes for genes and proteins, the discovery of new vectors for more efficient and specific targeting of inner ear cells, improved gene editing techniques, and the determination of the optimal therapeutic window and long-term effects of gene therapy.

The Auditory Hair Cells and Hearing in Mammals: Highly Specialized Needs, With Major Consequences

The inner ear comprises the cochlea, the sensory organ for hearing, and the vestibule, the organ responsible for balance (Figure 13.1a–c). Our ability to hear and communicate relies on the specialized functions carried out by various structures and cells within the cochlea, some of which are specific to mammals. These structures include the three fluid-filled canals, the hearing organ in the *scala media*, containing the *stria vascularis*, the basilar membrane, the tectorial membrane, the inner and outer hair cells (OHCs), and the associated neurons and supporting cells (Figure 13.1c). Throughout millions of years of evolution, our ears have developed a highly specialized architecture, with the appearance over time of new compartments (outer ear, middle ear, and cochlea), new structures (e.g., basilar membrane), and further specialization of the existing mechanosensitive

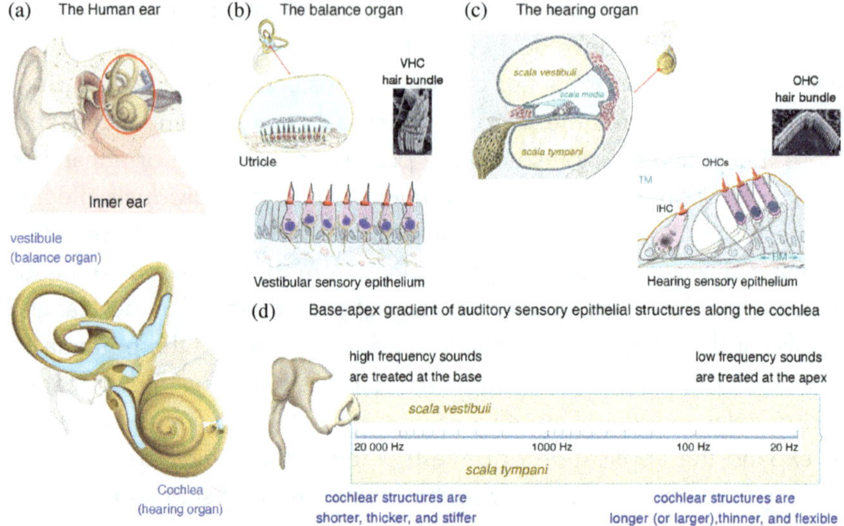

Fig. 13.1 **(a)** Anatomy of the human ear, depicting the inner ear composition, **(b)** balance and **(c)** hearing organ architecture, and **(d)** cochlear tonotopic organization. **(a)** The inner ear comprises the vestibule (balance organs), which detects linear and angular accelera tions, and the cochlea, which serves as the hearing organ, detecting sound waves. **(b)** In the balance organ, such as the utricle, body movements are sensed through the motion of the apical hair bundles of vestibular hair cells (VHCs). **(c)** Sounds are transduced in the cochlea, which consists of three fluid-filled compartments with different ionic compositions: the *scala vestibuli* (perilymph), *scala media* (endolymph), and *scala tympani* (perilymph). Sound conversion into electrical signals occurs in the *scala media*, which houses the auditory sensory organ, the organ of Corti, which includes hair cells, associated innervation, and various supporting cell types. The mammalian auditory sensory organ contains two types of hair cells: a single row of inner hair cells (IHCs, the genuine sensory cells) and three rows of outer hair cells (OHCs), responsible for sound amplification. **(d)** Along the cochlea, the structural and physical properties of the hair cells, the underlying basilar membrane (BM), and the overlying tectorial membrane (TM) gradually change from the base to the apex. The cochlear base (consisting of shorter and stiffer cells) primarily perceives high-frequency tones (up to 20 kHz in humans), whereas the apex (comprised of longer and more flexible cells) detects low-frequency sounds (20 Hz in humans). Adapted with permission from Delmaghani and El-Amraoui[1] and Maudoux *et al.*[5]

sensory hair cells (see Figure 13.2).[5] Among inner ear hair cells, the OHCs are unique to mammals and play a role in amplifying sound stimulation. They are found in three rows, numbering between 9,000 and 12,000 cells. On the other hand, the inner hair cells (IHCs), organized in a single row of 3,000–3,500 cells, are the true sensory cells responsible for transmitting sensory information to the central nervous system.[1,5]

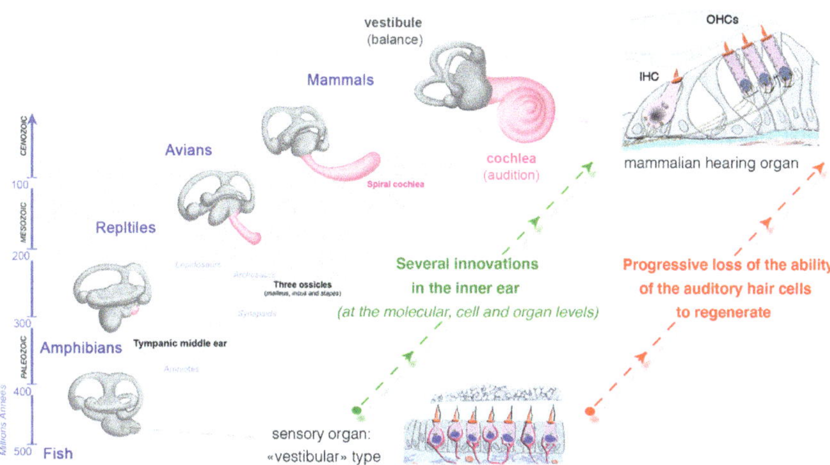

Fig. 13.2 Hearing is a relatively recent development in evolutionary history. While the organization and composition of the vestibular organ, crucial for gravity and balance detection, have remained largely unchanged throughout evolution, the auditory organ (depicted in purple) has undergone significant changes to adapt to the perception of acoustic stimuli. During evolution, species have progressively evolved to perceive higher frequency sounds. Amphibians can perceive sounds up to 1 kHz, avians up to 10 kHz, humans up to 20 kHz, and bats can detect frequencies as high as 160–200 kHz. These advancements were made possible through various innovations and specialization of existing structures within the hearing organs, including the emergence of outer hair cells (OHCs) unique to mammals. However, along with these changes, there has been a loss of capacity to regenerate auditory sensory cells in mammals. Unlike fish and amphibians, which retain the ability to produce hair cells throughout their lifetime, mammals lose this regenerative ability after embryonic development. Adapted with permission from Maudoux *et al.*[5]

The cochlea functions as a 'tonotopic organ' or a map where different regions, from the base to the apex, are tuned to specific pitches or tones (Figure 13.1d). This organization allows the brain to interpret, distinguish, and process different sounds. This precise mapping allows different frequencies to be processed separately, which enables us to distinguish and understand various speech sounds, perceive subtle nuances in music, and accurately discriminate between different frequencies in our environment. To achieve this, there's a gradual change in the molecular and structural architecture of the cells and structures that process sound along the auditory pathway. For instance, the physical and molecular properties of the hair cells and their adjacent supporting structures vary from base to apex of the cochlea (see Figure 13.1d).

In the basal region, the hair cells are shorter and stiffer, while in the apical region, they are longer and flexible (see Figure 13.1d).[1] The density and organization of neural connections between hair cells and auditory nerve fibers also gradually change along the cochlea, reflecting the tonotopic mapping and frequency selectivity. In humans, this tonotopic organization of the cochlea is vital for speech intelligibility. It enables us to hear frequencies ranging from 20 Hz to 20 kHz, with the apex of the cochlea analyzing low frequencies and the base analyzing high frequencies. Interestingly, during inner ear evolution (Figure 13.2), and for reasons that are still unclear, the ability of auditory hair cells to regenerate has been lost in mammals. Consequently, the number of hair cells and associated auditory neurons is predetermined before birth.[5] Since each region of the cochlea is essential, any loss or damage to these cells leads to hearing loss. Therefore, to fully restore hearing, treatment options must consider the spatial arrangement of sound frequencies in our auditory system.

Treating Hearing Loss: From Traditional Devices to Cutting-Edge Inner Ear Therapeutics

Currently, there is no cure for hearing loss. The available treatments include external hearing aids and cochlear implants. Hearing aids are recommended for mild-to-moderate hearing loss, while cochlear implants are used for severe-to-profound hearing loss. Cochlear implants bypass damaged hair cells by stimulating the auditory nerve with electrical impulses. However, these prosthetic devices only support speech frequencies (between 150 and 8,000 Hz) and provide limited sound discrimination compared to normal hearing. They also have limited effectiveness in noisy environments, and patient outcomes can vary significantly. Patients with cochlear implants must undergo a learning process to interpret sound. To improve auditory sensitivity and restore hearing more effectively, efforts are underway to develop complementary and additional treatment options. Various therapeutic approaches have been implemented and tested in the inner ear to evaluate their efficacy in restoring normal structure and function.

Pharmacological Therapy

Many studies are focused on identifying molecules with protective or reparative effects on sensory cells and/or auditory neurons. In clinical practice, several drugs, such as corticosteroids (e.g., prednisone, prednisolone, and dexamethasone), are used through oral or trans-tympanic applications. Some of these drugs may be effective when applied within a short time window before permanent sensorineural damage occurs. However, there is considerable variability in terms of efficacy and hearing improvement after treatment.[6]

Cell Therapy

Since the discovery of stem cells and their ability to repair damaged tissues, significant progress has been made in establishing protocols for controlled differentiation of stem cells into different types of inner ear cells, including hair cells, supporting cells, and neural cells.[7] These regenerative studies not only provide insights into the molecular and cellular mechanisms underlying hearing loss but also serve as cellular models for various hearing impairments. Cultivating cells in a three-dimensional environment has enabled the production of inner ear organoids (mini-ears) that closely resemble the intricate architecture and cellular composition of the inner ear. These organoids provide better models for studying inner ear development, disease mechanisms, and potential therapies. They also offer an efficient and cost-effective platform for drug discovery,[7,8] facilitating the identification of components that promote hair cell regeneration and protect against damage to hair cells and associated neurons.

Gene Therapy

Gene therapy is an innovative medical approach that has evolved to treat genetic diseases. The classical approach in gene therapy involves delivering a healthy gene into the cells expressing the disease. The delivered healthy genes can replace or supplement the faulty genes responsible for the disease. The therapeutic intervention can be designed to achieve a transient or permanent therapeutic effect for any type of gene and any type of cell. The goal is to correct the underlying genetic problem, helping the cells function properly. To achieve this goal, the delivery vectors play a crucial role in transporting healthy genes into the target cells. They are usually modified viruses that are made to be safe and harmless for our bodies. Each vector can target specific organ and specific cell types. Therefore, the choice of the type of vector for a given gene therapy will depend on its ability to target the right disease-expressing cells. The engineered or modified viruses or vectors act as delivery trucks that protect and deliver the genetic material to the correct location within the cells that contain the dysfunctional or missing gene. Once inside the cell, the genetic material provides all necessary instructions allowing the cell to function properly.

The chosen strategy for gene therapy can vary depending on the nature of the causal gene and the form and mode of transmission of the deafness. Individuals inherit two alleles for each gene, one from each parent. The gene replacement approach (Figure 13.3a), where a functional copy of the deficient gene is delivered directly to the target cells or reconstituted within them, is generally used to treat diseases with recessive transmission (both copies of the gene, called alleles and inherited from the father and mother, are dysfunctional) and loss-of-function dominant transmission, where the mutated copy of the gene causes a loss of function in the defective protein. In diseases with dominant transmission, the target cells often possess one functional copy and one mutated allele, which acts as a 'dominant negative' variant, interfering with normal allele function. The desired treatment involves removing the mutated variant to mitigate its detrimental impact on the functional allele. Gene editing strategies (Figure 13.3a) offer precise and specific targeting of disease-causing genes in such cases. These strategies can remove or silence the defective gene copy or correct the mutation and repair the faulty gene or allele. In the following sections, we will discuss recent successful endeavors in correcting hearing and/or vestibular disorders in more detail.

Moving Towards Corrective Therapies for Inner Ear Disorders: The Promises of Gene Therapy Research

Gene therapy research has shown promising results in the treatment of certain forms of blindness, raising hopes that similar therapeutic interventions could restore vestibular and auditory functions. Successful clinical

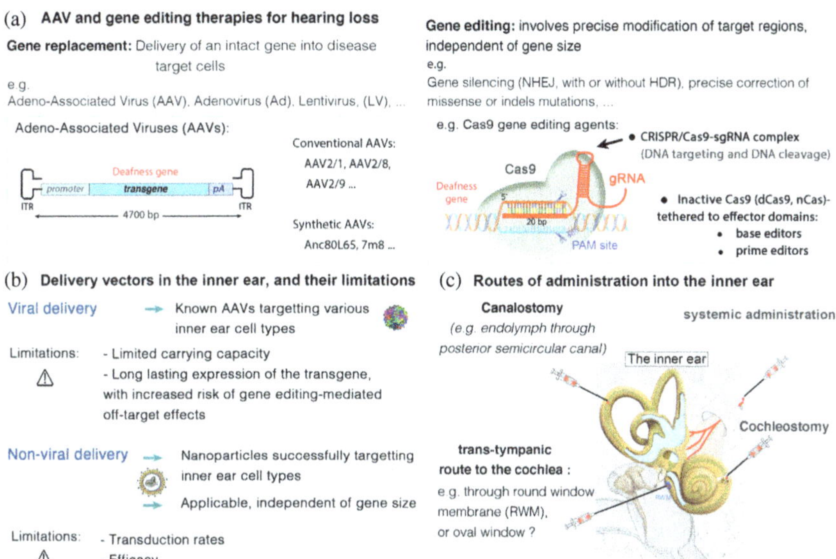

Fig. 13.3 Various therapeutic approaches are used to treat hearing loss. **(a)** Right panels: gene replacement (or supplementation) involves delivering a desired gene into target cells using vectors, replacing a defective gene or supplementing a therapeutic gene. Adeno-associated viruses (AAVs) are promising viral vectors used in clinical trials for rare diseases. However, their cargo capacity is limited to 5 kilobases, including promoter region, the transgene (~4.7 kilobases), and polyA 3 'region, between the two inverted terminal repeats (ITRs). Left panels: mutation-specific approaches use RNA/DNA gene editing strategies to modify gene sequences precisely, by removing, adding, or altering specific regions of the targeted gene. Applied strategies include anti-sense oligonucleotide (ASO), RNA interference, and the CRISPR/Cas9 system. Conventional Cas9 employs guide RNAs to direct Cas9 endonucleases to cut and repair specific regions, while base or prime editors have the potential to correct pathogenic mutations without disrupting the target gene. **(b)** Delivery strategies in the inner ear, using viral or non-viral vectors, have limitations. AAV-based gene replacement faces cargo capacity, tissue-specific targeting, and immune response challenges. CRISPR gene editing has off-target effects, HDR efficiency, and delivery difficulties to specific cells. Overcoming these limitations is crucial for maximizing CRISPR technology's potential in gene editing. **(c)** The main routes of administration in the inner ear include intracochlear delivery via the round window membrane (RWM), canalostomy through the posterior semicircular canal, and cochleostomy into the scala media. Other alternatives can be used, such as injection through the vestibular utricle, systemic application crossing the blood-labyrinth barrier, and middle ear delivery through diffusion via the round window. Adapted with permission from Botto *et al.*[3]

trials using gene replacement therapy in humans have been conducted to treat leber congenital amerosis (LCA) and choroideremia, among other retinal dystrophies.[3]

Gene Replacement Therapies

Adeno-associated virus (AAV) vectors have emerged as the most promising viral vectors for *in vivo* gene therapy in the ear due to their non-pathogenic and non-immunogenic nature, as well as their efficient targeting of inner ear cell types.[1,4] Due to their unique viral properties, each type of AAV vector (or serotype) exhibits a preference or affinity for infecting specific types of cells or tissues in the body, referred to as tropism. Over the recent years, researchers have harnessed the tropism of various AAV vectors to enhance the specificity and efficiency of gene delivery to the intended target cells in the inner ear (Figure 13.3a). The groundwork for using this approach in the ear was established in a mouse model of congenital deafness caused by a defect in the Vglut3 protein, a glutamate transporter expressed in IHCs.[9] For example, the transfer of AAV vectors of serotype 1 (AAV1) carrying the functional Vglut3 gene through the round window restored hearing to almost normal levels in the mouse model. Numerous studies using various models of deafness have since confirmed the efficacy of AAV-mediated gene supplementation for correcting inner ear defects (see Table 13.1, refer to Delmaghani and El-Amraoui,[1] Askew and Chien,[2] Botto *et al.*,[3] and Lahlou *et al.*[4] for more details). Variable degrees of hearing restoration have been reported in the treated mouse models, depending on the causal gene. However, restoration of vestibular function has often been complete and long-lasting. The success of gene therapy for hearing loss in these studies can be attributed, in part, to the high transfection efficiency of target cells, with most current AAVs transducing nearly 100% of IHCs.[1,4] These studies underscore the importance of identifying the appropriate therapeutic window for each type of deafness, as earlier gene delivery leads to more effective and sustained hearing restoration. Of note, AAV vectors have a limited capacity to carry genetic information, which is typically around 4.5–5.0 kilobase pairs (kb) of DNA (Figure 13.3a, b). To overcome the obstacle, dual AAV vectors were used to test possibility of splitting the therapeutic genetic material between 2 AAVs. This approach was successfully used in the inner ear, targeting two deafness genes, *OTOF*, encoding otoferlin[10,11] and *STRC*, encoding stereocilin.[12] The hearing restoration observed in studies targeting the OTOF gene has generated optimism for future gene therapy trials in humans.[4] Encouraged by these

Table 13.1 List of deafness genes for which gene therapy has been used to restore hearing (and balance).

Used therapeutic strategy	Gene (deafness)/OMIM number	Mouse model
	Gene replacement/gene supplementation	
Single AAV	VGLUT3 (DFNA25)/**607557**	$Vglut3^{-/-}$
	GJB6 (DFNB1)/**604418**	$Gjb6^{-/-}$
	GJB2 (DFNB1)/**121011**	*Foxg1-cCx26 KO*
	MSRB3 (DFNB74)/**613719**	$MsrB3^{-/-}$
	TMC1 (DFNB7/11)/**606706**	$Tmc1^{Bth/+}$
	TMC1 (DFNA36)/**606706**	$Tmc1^{Bth/+}$
	PJVK (DFNB59)/**610219**	$Pjvk^{-/-}$
	LHFPL5 (DFNB67)/**609427**	$Lhflp5^{-/-}$
	USH1C (Usher type 1C)/**605242**	*Ush1c* c.216G > A KI
	USH1G (Usher type 1G)/**607696**	$Ush1g^{-/-}$
	WHRN (Usher type 2D)/**607928**	$Whrn^{wi/wi}$
	CLRN1 (Usher type 3)/**606397**	*cClrn1* KO and $Clrn1^{-/-}$
	PCDH15 (DFNB23)/**605514**	$Pcdh15^{av3j}$
	SYNE4/**615535**	$Syne4^{-/-}$
	KCNQ1 (Jervell and Lange-Nielsen)/**607542**	$Kcnq1^{-/-}$
	TMPRSS3 (DFNB8)/**605511**	$Tmprss3^{A306T/A306T}$
Dual AAVs	OTOF (DFNB9)/**603681**	$Otof^{-/-}$
	STRC (DFNB16)/**606440**	$Strc^{-/-}$
	RNA therapies	
Anti-sense oligonucleotides	USH1C (Usher type 1C)/**605242**	*Ush1c* c.216G > A KI
RNA interference	GJB2 (DFNB1)/**121011**	*WT mice expressing* $pGJB2^{R75W}$*-eGFP*
	CRISPR-mediated gene editing	
CRISPR-Cas9	TMC1 (DFNA36)/**606706**	$Tmc1^{Bth/+}$
CRISPR-Cas9	ATP2B2, or PMCA2 (DFNA82)/**108733**	$Atp2b2^{Obl/+}$
CRISPR-Cas9	KCNQ4 (DFNA2)/**603537**	$Kcnq4^{-/-}$
CRISPR-Cas9	PCDH15 (DFNB23)/**605514**	$Pcdh15^{av3j}$
CRISPR-Cas9	MYO6 (DFNA22)/**600970**	$Myo6^{WT/C442Y}$
Base editing	TMC1 (DFNB7/11)/**606706**	$Tmc1^{Y182C/Y182C}$

Refer to Delmaghani and El-Amraoui,[1] Askew and Chien,[2] Botto *et al.*,[3] and Lahlou *et al.*[4] for more details, and to the OMIM number for detailed information on the defective gene, and reference to the causal disease and related animal models.

findings, pharmaceutical companies are actively engaged in the development of gene therapy products specifically designed for individuals that carry mutations in the OTOF gene, offering hope for potential therapeutic interventions in the near future.

Genome Editing to Treat Specific Deafness Mutations

In certain cases of recurrent mutations, targeted molecular approaches can be used to correct specific regions of the defective gene. Here are some recent examples:

Anti-sense oligonucleotides

Anti-sense oligonucleotides (ASOs) are small nucleotide sequences that can block defective splicing of a disease gene. Splicing is a cellular process that removes noncoding segments (introns) from a gene's transcript and joins together the coding segments (exons) to create a functional messenger RNA (mRNA) molecule for protein production. ASOs can be designed to promote correct splicing of targeted messenger RNA, leading to the production of a normal protein. This approach was successfully employed to bypass a common mutation causing Usher syndrome, an inherited disorder causing deafness and blindness.[13] For example, a frequent mutation in the USH1C gene that leads to profound deafness in mice was targeted using ASOs. Lentz *et al.* identified an ASO sequence that corrected the splicing and restored auditory and vestibular functions, increased wild-type protein levels, and restored the morphology of hair cell bundles.[14] ASOs hold potential for treating other types of deafness-causing mutations.[14,15]

RNA interference

This approach was used in a model of DFNA3, a form of dominant transmission deafness caused by a mutation in the connexin-26 gene. A gelatin product containing liposomes with specific RNA interference (RNAi) for the mutated allele of connexin-26 was applied to the round window membrane in the model. The RNAi reduced the expression of the mutated allele by 70% and halted the progression of hearing loss without affecting the healthy allele.[16] This demonstrates the potential of RNAi for *in vivo* treatment of genetic deafness caused by dominant negative effects.

CRISPR/Cas9 genome editing

The development of genome editing tools like CRISPR/Cas9 provides efficient and precise ways to modify DNA at specific locations for long-lasting treatment (Figure 13.3a). Recent studies have used this approach to correct causal mutations that lead to hearing loss.[1,3] Selected guide RNAs were used to correct mutations in genes such as *ATB2B2* (PMCA2), *TMC1*, *MYO6*, and *KCNQ4 in vitro* and then delivered via injection to the inner ear of corresponding mouse models (see Table 13.1). These studies showed significant auditory recovery, improved cell survival, and preservation of associated innervation in the mouse models.[17] However, concerns about the specificity of nucleases and *in vivo* delivery methods still needs to be addressed.[1–4]

These findings demonstrate the potential of gene editing approaches for *in vivo* treatment of genetic deafness with dominant negative effects. Function's alteration, repression, activation, and correction of targeted genes can be precisely designed with the use of the gene editing new tools (Figure 13.3a). Further research is required to enhance their efficacy, understand the mechanisms of ASOs and nucleases, and investigate their safety and potential off-target effects (see Figure 13.3b).

'Gene-Independent' Approaches as a Common Strategy for Several Forms of Deafness

Given the large number of genes involved in deafness, correcting each individual defect is a challenging task in the short or medium term. Therefore, gene-independent therapies that can be applied to multiple forms of deafness, whether inherited or acquired, hold promise for preserving or restoring functional auditory structures. For more comprehensive information, refer to recent reviews.[1–4]

Regeneration of hair cells

One approach focuses on regenerating or replacing defective hair cells to protect and prevent the deterioration of hearing. A strategy involves the overexpression of a transcription factor called Math1. Transcription factors act as molecular switches that help control the activity of genes within cells, influencing how cell develop and function. Previous work has demonstrated the ability of Math1 (also called atonal) to trigger and coordinate the expression of genes that convert supporting cells into new hair cells in the cochlea. Encouraging results, including partial restoration of hearing thresholds, have been observed in studies conducted on mice and guinea pigs. The world's first gene therapy trial for hearing loss, which aimed to test the safety of delivering an adenovirus-Math1 to patients via a trans-tympanic approach (NCT02132130), has recently been completed. However, no follow-up action has been proposed yet. It should be noted that injecting Math1 at later stages in animals has shown limited effectiveness, and this approach cannot be currently used for genetically caused deafness without addressing the underlying genetic mutation.

Protection of hearing through local therapies

Another promising approach focuses on the survival pathways of hair cells and associated neurons, which can be affected by genetic anomalies, noise exposure, or ototoxic agents (substances or medications) that can cause damage to the structures of the ear, specifically the sensory cells responsible for hearing and balance. Efforts have been directed towards gene transfer of growth factors or mitotic agents that can activate these survival pathways in hair cells and neurons. The goal is to preserve as many neurons as possible and promote their regrowth to enhance neural transmission and auditory performance. Recent studies utilizing molecules like NT3 have demonstrated protective effects in animal models, limiting the impact of cochlear synaptopathies that affect the connections or synapses between the sensory hair cells and the auditory nerve fibers.[18] However, further detailed studies in animal models are necessary before considering their application in humans.

From Preclinical Models to Humans: The Multiple Challenges of Inner Ear Therapeutics

Gene therapies have shown promising potential for the prevention and treatment of hearing impairment and vestibular defects. While still in the early stages of development, the success of inner ear therapeutics in animal models instills hope for their future application in clinical settings. Continuous research and development efforts will enable researchers to optimize gene therapy for inner ear disorders and overcome the challenges associated with their translation into clinical practice.

Avenues for Hair Cell Regeneration

Many studies aim to regenerate or replace defective hair cells to protect against or prevent hearing loss. *In vitro* and animal studies have yielded promising results with the overexpression of the Math1 transcription factor. However, questions remain regarding Math1's ability to produce hair cells at the appropriate stage of development in a consistent manner, as well as the long-term effectiveness of the Math1 pathway. Other avenues for regeneration exist in non-mammalian vertebrates, but their identification and the potential for their reactivation in the mammalian ear, particularly in an adult non-permissive environment, need further exploration. It should be noted that this strategy may not be applicable to genetic hearing loss without simultaneous correction of the underlying mutation.

Reproduction and Maintenance of Cochlear Tonotopy

Restoring normal hearing after hearing loss requires the preservation of the tonotopic organization of the mature cochlea, which is established during embryonic development. Therapeutic approaches must ensure that repaired or newly differentiated cells possess properties consistent with their position along the cochlea and can effectively establish connections with support cells and innervating neurons. Reestablishing the precise mapping of cochlear tonotopy in a defective cochlea at mature stages is essential for achieving normal speech intelligibility and restoring the ability to perceive subtle nuances in music. It also enables accurate discrimination between different frequencies in our environment.

Choice of Vectors, Target Cells, and Administration Routes

Delivering therapeutic agents to the inner ear is challenging due to its specialized architecture and fluid-filled spaces (see Figure 13.3c). The selection of appropriate vectors plays a critical role in the success of gene therapy, and overcoming the obstacles associated with inner ear access is crucial for ongoing therapeutic developments, whether genetic, cellular, or pharmacological. AAV vectors have been the most successful vector in gene replacement studies, with different serotypes exhibiting specific tropism for targeting specific cells. However, AAVs have limitations in terms of their capacity to accommodate large genes (>4,500 base pairs) (Figure 13.3a, b).[1,4] Efforts are being made to explore the potential of other viruses with larger packaging capacities, such as lentiviruses and adenoviruses, to target inner ear cell types. However, the use of these viruses in clinical settings still carries the risk of triggering an immune response. Novel synthetic AAV vectors are being designed and tested to improve cellular targeting, and alternative routes of administration (e.g., diffusion through the round window membrane, direct intracochlear injection, cochleostomy, semicircular canals, and systemic delivery) are being explored (Figure 13.3c).[1–4] Additionally, non-viral vectors such as liposomes, metallic and polymeric nanoparticles, and gels, which offer high drug/gene-loading capacity and efficient absorption in the inner ear, are also being developed to enhance targeting efficiency (Figure 13.3b). Ongoing efforts to expand the range of efficient and safe delivery methods are critical for identifying suitable vectors capable of expressing therapeutic agents and targeting the appropriate cells based on the chosen route and timing of delivery.

Personalized Hearing Medicine

The identification of specific genes responsible for hearing loss has led to a better understanding of the inner ear's anatomy and physiology, opening the door to personalized medicine for hearing loss.[1–4] The diverse genetic and phenotypic forms of hearing loss necessitate the development of tailored treatment solutions. To evaluate treatment efficacy in humans, precise and accurate clinical endpoints need to be identified based on the causal gene, leading to the development of personalized therapies. These targeted therapies should be adapted to the causal agent and defective mechanisms, the target cell type (hair cells, supporting cells, or neurons), the degree and onset of hearing impairment, and the intended goal of treatment (protection, prevention, restoration, or replacement of damaged cells). Evaluation of therapy effectiveness and safety should be conducted within a time window applicable to humans, considering the natural history of the disease in human patients. The safety of surgery, gene delivery vector, and therapeutic transgene must also be evaluated before administering gene therapy to humans. Assessing the risks associated with potential adverse effects on the immune system caused by the therapeutic intervention is important. These effects can include unwanted immune reactions, immune system dysfunction, or excessive inflammation that even damage inner ear cells and organs.

In conclusion, the personalized hearing medicine offers exciting prospects for individuals with hearing loss. With advancements in our understanding of the inner ear's pathology and the development of tailored therapies, it is becoming increasingly feasible to address the diverse causes of deafness. The future success of cochlear gene therapy will depend on achieving results that are at least as good as those of cochlear implants. While challenges remain, the continued efforts and recent success in animal models are promising. As Louis Pasteur once said, 'Chance only favors the prepared mind.' Continued research and collaboration across disciplines, with effective cooperation among scientists, clinicians, audiologists, and other stakeholders in the inner ear field will be instrumental in optimizing inner ear therapeutics, overcoming existing challenges, and ultimately translating these advancements into effective clinical interventions that can restore and improve hearing function in patients.

Acknowledgements

The work in the authors' laboratories is funded by the French National Research Agency (ANR), as part of the second 'Investissements d'Avenir' program (light4deaf, ANR-15-RHUS-0001), ANR-HearInNoise (ANR-17-CE16-0017), EuroNanoMed-NanoEar (ANR-21-ENM3-0003-04), and Fondation Pour l'Audition (FPA-19-Stg). The support provided to the Institut de l'Audition by Fondation Pour l'Audition is acknowledged and apologies to authors of other relevant work that was not cited here due to space constraints.

References

1. Delmaghani S, El-Amraoui A. (2020) Inner ear gene therapies take off: Current promises and future challenges. *J Clin Med* **9**(7):2309.
2. Askew C, Chien WW. (2020) Adeno-associated virus gene replacement for recessive inner ear dysfunction: Progress and challenges. *Hear Res* **394**:107947.
3. Botto C, Dalkara D, El-Amraoui A. (2021) Progress in gene editing tools and their potential for correcting mutations underlying hearing and vision loss. *Front Gene Edit* **3**:737632.
4. Lahlou G, Calvet C, Giorgi M, *et al.* (2023) Towards the clinical application of gene therapy for genetic inner ear diseases. *J Clin Med* **12**(3):1046.
5. Maudoux A, Vitry S, El-Amraoui A. (2022) Vestibular deficits in deafness: Clinical presentation, animal modeling and treatment solutions. *Front Neurol* **13**:816534.
6. Liu SS, Yang R. (2022) Inner ear drug delivery for sensorineural hearing loss: Current challenges and opportunities. *Front Neurosci* **16**:867453.
7. Koehler KR, Nie J, Longworth-Mills E, *et al.* (2017) Generation of inner ear organoids containing functional hair cells from human pluripotent stem cells. *Nat Biotechnol* **35**:583–9.
8. Roccio M, Edge ASB. (2019) Inner ear organoids: New tools to understand neurosensory cell development, degeneration and regeneration. *Development* **146**(17):dev177188.
9. Akil O, Seal RP, Burke K, *et al.* (2012) Restoration of hearing in the VGLUT3 knockout mouse using virally mediated gene therapy. *Neuron* **75**(2):283–93.
10. Al-Moyed H, Cepeda AP, Jung S, *et al.* (2019) A dual-AAV approach restores fast exocytosis and partially rescues auditory function in deaf otoferlin knock-out mice. *EMBO Mol Med* **11**(1):e9396.
11. Akil O, Dyka F, Calvet C, *et al.* (2019) Dual AAV-mediated gene therapy restores hearing in a DFNB9 mouse model. *Proc Natl Acad Sci U S A* **116**(10):4496–501.
12. Shubina-Oleinik O, Nist-Lund C, French C, *et al.* (2021) Dual-vector gene therapy restores cochlear amplification and auditory sensitivity in a mouse model of DFNB16 hearing loss. *Sci Adv* **7**(51):eabi7629.
13. Delmaghani S, El-Amraoui A. (2022) The genetic and phenotypic landscapes of Usher syndrome: From disease mechanisms to a new classification. *Hum Genet* **141**(3–4):709–35.

14. Lentz JJ, Jodelka FM, Hinrich AJ, *et al.* (2013) Rescue of hearing and vestibular function by antisense oligonucleotides in a mouse model of human deafness. *Nat Med* **19**(3):345–50.
15. Wang L, Kempton JB, Jiang H, *et al.* (2020) Fetal antisense oligonucleotide therapy for congenital deafness and vestibular dysfunction. *Nucleic Acids Res* **48**(9):5065–80.
16. Maeda Y, Sheffield AM, Smith RJH. (2009) Therapeutic regulation of gene expression in the inner ear using RNA interference. *Adv Otorhinolaryngol* **66**:13–36.
17. Yeh WH, Shubina-Oleinik O, Levy JM, *et al.* (2020) *In vivo* base editing restores sensory transduction and transiently improves auditory function in a mouse model of recessive deafness. *Sci Transl Med* 12(546):eaay9101.
18. Cassinotti LR, Ji L, Borges BC, *et al.* (2022) Cochlear Neurotrophin-3 overexpression at mid-life prevents age-related inner hair cell synaptopathy and slows age-related hearing loss. *Aging Cell* **21**(10):e13708.

14 Robotic Ear Surgery

C. Cooper Munhall, MD[1]; Katherine E. Riojas, PhD[2];
Robert F. Labadie, MD, PhD[1]

Abstract

Robots have allowed for great advances in safety, efficiency, and cost-saving measures across many fields. Although robotic systems in surgery can offer similar benefits, implementation in healthcare settings is accompanied by stringent legislative and patient safety barriers. There are several types of robotic systems being used, tested, or developed for applications in ear surgery. This chapter discusses three main types of robotic surgical systems: 1 — collaborative/guide; 2 — teleoperated; and 3 — autonomous. While each of these systems has various benefits and limitations, they all offer the potential to augment or optimize various otologic surgical techniques. We focus on two clinical applications within ear surgery especially suited for robotic incorporation: surgical drilling and insertion of cochlear implant (CI) electrode arrays. Robotic systems for both drilling (minimally invasive tunneled techniques and bulk drilling applications) and CI electrode insertion have been developed to improve current techniques and are discussed throughout this chapter.

Introduction

The development of robots has allowed for stark changes to many fields (e.g., automation in industrial manufacturing, agriculture, and food production), and their utilization has often led to improved safety, efficiency,

---

Corresponding Author: Robert F. Labadie MD, PhD

[1] Department of Otolaryngology — Head and Neck Surgery, Medical University of South Carolina, Charleston, SC, United States.

[2] Department of Mechanical Engineering, Vanderbilt University, Nashville, TN, United States.

and cost-saving measures. In each field, the introduction and widespread utilization of robotic elements has required both technological innovation as well as social adoption. While incorporation of robotic elements into healthcare and surgical practice is constrained by similar factors, it also faces unique limitations, chief among them being patient safety concerns. Despite the difficulties faced by robotic developers attempting to break into this space, there are already several robots approved for use in operating rooms around the world.

Within otolaryngology, the most recognizable robot in use is likely the da Vinci surgical system created by Intuitive Surgical. This surgical system was first introduced in the late 1990s, received FDA clearance in 2000, and has been implemented across several surgical specialties. The da Vinci surgical system offers advantages primarily in visualization and surgical maneuverability, which are helpful for difficult-to-access areas such as the base of tongue. Mechanical elements of the system include wristed instruments that mirror typical surgical motions and a close-up 3D-HD view of the anatomy, both of which are designed primarily to enhance traditional surgical methods. This device is currently used within otolaryngology mainly for transoral robotic surgery (TORS) in the surgical resection of various oral cavity/oropharyngeal cancers. Locations deep within the oral cavity can significantly limit surgical maneuverability using traditional approaches, and the increased length and surgical dexterity provided by this system can allow for unparalleled access without such invasive measures as splitting the jaw. While the role of the da Vinci surgical system is more clear-cut in areas of otolaryngology such as base of tongue resections, its potential role in ear surgery has yet to be established with cadaveric studies demonstrating feasibility but limited potential benefit, given that the original and subsequent models of the da Vinci surgical system (models Si, X, and Xi) were designed for multiple-port laparoscopic surgery.[1] For narrow-field surgery, such as middle ear access, a miniaturized version of the newer da Vinci single port (SP) system may have utility.

While many robotic applications in ear surgery are still in their infancy, there are many implementations which may be able to augment or optimize surgical techniques in otology and neurotology. The use of robots within the surgical environment raises dichotomous questions about patient safety, both in their potential ability to help surgeons avoid dangerous situations intraoperatively and in their potential to malfunction and lead to harm. The perceived benefits of surgical robots include optimized surgical visualization, minimally invasive techniques, increased surgical efficiency, and the elimination of various human physical limitations, among others. Ultimately, clinicians and patients alike may hope for improved surgical outcomes through the implementation of robotic technology. In this chapter discussing the current state of robotic ear surgery, we must first define types of robotic systems. As previously done, in this chapter we will separate robots in ear surgery based on their role within the surgeon–device–patient interaction with 'end-effector' defined as the surgical instrument in contact with the patient.[2]

— Collaborative robot/guide — The surgeon directly actuates the end-effector(s). The robot/guide passively or actively constrains and potentially impacts surgical motions.
— Teleoperated robot — The surgeon remotely controls the end-effector(s) during the surgery [i.e., surgeon's motions are mapped to end-effector(s) motions with potential modification (i.e., tremor reduction, scaling)].
— Autonomous robot — The end-effector interacts with the patient without active input from the surgeon, with the surgeon overseeing the robot. Note that the surgeon must initiate such autonomous robotic systems (perhaps with a button push/hold) and monitors the operative progression, intervening if necessary.

Clinical Implementations

While not necessarily inherent to surgical robotic systems themselves, the necessity for linking robotic systems discussed throughout this chapter to patient anatomy is a key component in successful and safe clinical integration. Currently, there are two primary methods by which such anatomical linking has been established: image-guidance systems and physically linked systems through rigid attachment to the skull. Among image-guidance systems, only infrared tracking has been consistently used for implementation of surgical robotic systems. Limitations of this image-guidance modality include the necessity for clear line-of-sight tracking, which can be obscured with alterations in the surgical field such as bone dust, irrigation, or bleeding.

The advantages are its high tracking accuracy to a level of microscopic detail required in ear surgery. While electromagnetic tracking systems do not rely on line-of-sight and are thus unimpeded by visual disturbances to the surgical field, they currently lack the level of tracking accuracy necessary to safely link robotic systems to patient anatomy. Rigid skull fixation has been heavily utilized within the field of neurosurgery and provides for extremely accurate tracking at the cost of a more invasive surgical procedure. The rest of this chapter will discuss various clinical applications within ear surgery that surgical robots have been or could be used to improve patient outcomes, safety, or surgical efficiency.

Surgical Drilling

Drilling is a key component of most otologic procedures allowing access to critical structures within the middle or inner ear. Many ear surgeries involve bulk drilling of the mastoid bone while others require precision small-scale drilling for formation of a stapedotomy or cochleostomy. A variety of robotic surgical systems may have potential application for these specific purposes, with unique contributions by robotic type.

Collaborative/guide

Perhaps the simplest robotic system to appreciate is the collaborative surgical robot or guide. Included within this category are frames/templates that align a surgical instrument to unique patient anatomy along a specific trajectory. Such systems have been utilized for neurosurgical procedures since the 1970s, initially with rigid, stereotactic N-frames and then robotic arms to obtain minimally invasive intracranial biopsies and perform other procedures requiring highly accurate intracranial localization.[3,4] Within ear surgery, similar applications utilizing an individualized microstereotactic frame have been reported to access the cochlea in a minimally invasive fashion. Labadie *et al.* successfully demonstrated such a technique in nine patients, using a customized microstereotactic frame to access the cochlea by drilling a narrow tunnel along a pre-planned trajectory from the surface of the mastoid through the facial recess.[5] Minimally invasive approaches utilizing such technology may improve patient outcomes regarding hospital length of stay and analgesic requirements along with increased surgical efficiency.

Slightly more involved collaborative robots have been employed to limit surgical motions in patient-specific 'no-fly zones' to prevent damage to critical structures or surrounding healthy tissue. While the surgeon can drill normally within the predetermined safe boundary, surgical motion outside this area is prevented by robotic systems using active braking with motors or passive braking with electromagnets.[6,7] Such 'no-fly zones' may be particularly useful within surgical education, allowing for more expanded surgical involvement for trainees while providing a protective barrier to maximize patient safety. Robotically enforced surgical boundaries may also find application in cases with complicated or atypical patient anatomy identified and mapped preoperatively, helping provide indication of danger zones that would be more readily identified and avoided in typical patients.

Teleoperated

While the previously mentioned da Vinci surgical system is perhaps the most widely utilized robotic system within otolaryngology, teleoperated systems have not yet experienced widespread clinical utilization within ear surgery. There are several potential benefits of teleoperated systems within the context of surgical drilling, with similar potential utility in establishing 'no-fly zones,' force perception thresholds surpassing human abilities, and minimization of tremor, among other possible features. RobOtol is the only teleoperated robotic system currently approved for clinical use and is commercially available in the European Union with C-E mark approval. This teleoperated system, designed in Paris, France, at the Pierre and Marie Curie University, consists of a platform opposite the surgeon with two effector arms controlled by the surgeon via an interface either with a computer mouse or with a stylus. This teleoperated system allows anatomical scaling of various surgical motions, to allow for gross movements while drilling versus more limited movement for microsurgical motions. Clinical utilizations described initially have focused on simple tasks to practice clinical integration and familiarity with system functionality. In addition to more gross utilization of RobOtol in drilling of the mastoid, it could have potential utility in drilling for stapedotomy or cochleostomy creation. While damage to the internal endosteum of the labyrinth is a possibility, even with the human threshold for force detection, a teleoperated system such as RobOtol paired with force perception capabilities could significantly limit such trauma. Such utilization has not yet been demonstrated clinically, although an uncooked egg served as a surrogate by researchers at Birmingham University in the United Kingdom.[8] Their device was able to successfully drill through the outer shell of an uncooked egg without disrupting the inner membrane lining the shell. It stands to reason that teleoperated systems could similarly demonstrate such precision and avoidance of traumatic drilling for cochleostomy and stapedotomy formation.

Autonomous

Autonomous robots may be more in-line with what people typically envision robots to be, and there are a myriad of potential benefits to their involvement in ear surgery. Surgical drilling of the mastoid is an area within ear surgery that autonomous or semi-autonomous robots have legitimate potential, both in cochlear access using minimally invasive tunnelling techniques or drilling larger regions of the mastoid to either obliterate disease and/or provide access (e.g., chronic mastoiditis, access to inner ear). Several groups have already demonstrated tunneled approaches to the cochlea using an autonomous industrial arm robot as well as a custom-built autonomous robotic system called the HEARO, both of which employ image-guidance techniques for navigation.[9,11] The HEARO surgical robot for cochlear implant (CI) surgery has received certification mark (CE) approval and is now being used in multiple clinical locations throughout Europe. This autonomous robotic system includes a multi-articulated arm and utilized preoperative imaging to identify a safe trajectory for minimally invasive access to the cochlea. Chief among the critical structures at risk during ear surgery and particularly during drilling is the facial nerve, and the HEARO employs several strategies to avoid damaging it including using the drill as a facial nerve stimulator to continuously monitor its functional status. In addition to drilling of the mastoid, the HEARO may hold future utility in preserving the internal endosteum in cochleostomy if paired with force perception capabilities.

In addition to tunnelling for cochlear access and cochleostomy/stapedotomy formation, more involved surgical drilling approaches have been demonstrated with autonomous or semi-autonomous robotic systems. A full mastoidectomy was initially demonstrated via an autonomous robotic system equipped with image-guidance software more than a decade ago.[12] Modifications made by Danilchenko *et al.* to an industrial robotic arm facilitated wielding of a surgical drill tracked via infrared technology to successfully allow safe and complete drilling of the mastoid. Meanwhile, trans-labyrinthine approaches to the internal auditory canal (IAC) have been drilled in cadavers using a lightweight, autonomous robot with expanded surgical maneuverability.[13] This robot was utilized to perform the majority of drilling without damage to vital anatomy in all six cadaveric specimens, removing more than 95% of the volume of bone required for the approach. A trans-labyrinthine approach was similarly achieved by another group using rigid fixation to a cadaver and a computer-aided surgical machining system.[14] Autonomous surgical robots used in drilling the majority of mastoids or approaches to the IAC might allow for increased surgical efficiency and direct involvement of the surgeon on end effectors only at critical portions requiring skilled human surgical involvement.

Insertion of Electrode Array

Cochlear implant surgery has experienced many innovations in the design of implants, magnets, and electrode arrays leading to improved hearing outcomes for patients, which likely will expand the potential patient population. Standardization of techniques in CI surgery has been developed to improve hearing outcomes. However, at present, outcomes in residual hearing preservation and overall hearing are still highly variable which likely relates to the process of inserting the electrode array. Intracochlear trauma sustained during the insertion process could potentially be reduced using robotic technology with the ideal robotic insertion system offering slow continuous insertion, force detection below the threshold for intracochlear trauma, and programmable angle and depth of insertion based on individual patient anatomy, among other features. In this vein, we will discuss robots currently in use or under development as well as potential future applications within the previously defined robotic categories.

Collaborative/guide

The application of guide robotic systems in electrode insertion could potentially have similar utilization as microstereotactic frames or other such systems customized for individual patient anatomy. Such guides could allow for pre-determined optimal angle of insertion of the electrode array to help minimize intracochlear trauma. Collaborative tools could theoretically include force feedback paired mechanisms to limit insertional forces. Such collaborative or guide robotic systems for CI electrode array insertion have yet to be developed or implemented clinically.

Teleoperated

Teleoperated systems are ideally suited for force feedback mechanisms that do not rely on human input to minimize trauma during the insertion process. Efforts by Zhang *et al.* to incorporate such into the field of otologic surgery include a system that allows for force perception capabilities and haptic feedback while remotely steering an electrode array during insertion. The developers of the aforementioned RobOtol have also created an assistive insertion tool coupled with the RobOtol system which shows fewer and less sudden peaks of insertion forces.[15,16] Such teleoperated systems, known as master-slave systems in the robotics world, are likely to be a temporary step towards surgeons trusting and then ceding control to autonomous robots with autonomous robots offering the large advance of achieving suprahuman thresholds which will be necessary to consistently avoid intracochlear damage during electrode insertion.

Autonomous

Humans lack the ability to consistently detect rupture of the osseous spiral lamina and basilar membrane, which makes atraumatic insertion an ideal task for an autonomous robot.[17] With a pre-specified trajectory for the CI electrode array based on preoperative imaging, insertion becomes a much simpler task focused primarily on linear advancement, particularly so for straight, or 'lateral-wall,' arrays. Pre-curved, or 'perimodiolar,' electrode arrays involve slightly more attention with a stylet for advancement that must be stopped during initial insertion. An autonomous robotic system has been used to insert electrodes with several of these parameters in mind, allowing for linear advancement of the electrode and stoppage of the stylet. While at this stage in development, humans were, in some instances, able to perform electrode insertion better than the robot, the robotic system demonstrated consistently low insertion forces that are likely tied to fewer instances of traumatic insertion.[18,19] A slow insertion robotic tool, IotaMotion, has recently received FDA approval and shown to significantly reduce overall insertion force, force variability, and severe intracochlear trauma events in cadaveric temporal bones with clinical reports pending (NCT04577118).[20]

Conclusion

Many of the surgical robots discussed within this chapter have not been clinically implemented and may not be fully utilized for some time. Ultimately, technological breakthroughs in these systems that allow for significantly improved patient outcomes and/or cost-effectiveness compared with traditional ear surgery are likely prerequisites for widespread clinical adoption. Although the particularly stringent restrictions and regulations within healthcare regarding robotic implementation may hinder adoption, there are already a wide variety of robotic surgical systems being utilized within ear surgery for various procedures.

References

1. Liu WP, Azizian M, Sorger J, *et al.* (2014) Cadaveric feasibility study of da Vinci Si-assisted cochlear implant with augmented visual navigation for otologic surgery. *JAMA Otolaryngol Head Neck Surg* **140**(3):208–14.
2. Riojas KE, Labadie RF. (2020) Robotic ear surgery. *Otolaryngol Clin North Am* **53**(6):1065–75.
3. Brown RA. (1979) A stereotactic head frame for use with CT body scanners. *Invest Radiol* **14**(4):300–4.
4. Kwoh YS, Hou J, Jonckheere EA, Hayati S. (1988) A robot with improved absolute positioning accuracy for CT guided stereotactic brain surgery. *IEEE Trans Biomed Eng* **35**(2):153–60.
5. Labadie RF, Balachandran R, Noble JH, *et al.* (2014) Minimally invasive image-guided cochlear implantation surgery: First report of clinical implementation. *Laryngoscope* **124**(8):1915–22.

6. Yoo MH, Lee HS, Yang CJ, *et al.* (2017) A cadaver study of mastoidectomy using an image-guided human-robot collaborative control system. *Laryngoscope Investig Otolaryngol* **2**(5):208–14.
7. Lim H, Matsumoto N, Cho B, *et al.* (2016) Semi-manual mastoidectomy assisted by human-robot collaborative control — A temporal bone replica study. *Auris Nasus Larynx* **43**(2):161–5.
8. Coulson CJ, Assadi MZ, Taylor RP, *et al.* (2013) A smart micro-drill for cochleostomy formation: A comparison of cochlear disturbances with manual drilling and a human trial. *Cochlear Implants Int* **14**(2):98–106.
9. Majdani O, Rau TS, Baron S, *et al.* (2009) A robot-guided minimally invasive approach for cochlear implant surgery: Preliminary results of a temporal bone study. *Int J Comput Assist Radiol Surg* **4**(5):475–86.
10. Baron S, Eilers H, Munske B, *et al.* (2010) Percutaneous inner-ear access via an image-guided industrial robot system. *Proc Inst Mech Eng H* **224**(5):633–49.
11. Caversaccio M, Wimmer W, Anso J, *et al.* (2019) Robotic middle ear access for cochlear implantation: First in man. *PLoS One* **14**(8):e0220543.
12. Danilchenko A, Balachandran R, Toennies JL, *et al.* (2011) Robotic mastoidectomy. *Otol Neurotol* **32**(1):11–6.
13. Dillon NP, Balachandran R, Siebold MA, *et al.* (2017) Cadaveric testing of robot-assisted access to the internal auditory canal for vestibular schwannoma removal. *Otol Neurotol* **38**(3):441–7.
14. Couldwell WT, MacDonald JD, Thomas CL, *et al.* (2017) Computer-aided design/computer-aided manufacturing skull base drill. *Neurosurg Focus* **42**(5):E6.
15. Barriat S, Peigneux N, Duran U, *et al.* (2021) The use of a robot to insert an electrode array of cochlear implants in the cochlea: A feasibility study and preliminary results. *Audiol Neurootol* **26**(5):361–7.
16. Nguyen Y, Kazmitcheff G, De Seta D, *et al.* (2014) Definition of metrics to evaluate cochlear array insertion forces performed with forceps, insertion tool, or motorized tool in temporal bone specimens. *Biomed Res Int* **2014**:532570.
17. Kratchman LB, Schuster D, Dietrich MS, *et al.* (2016) Force perception thresholds in cochlear implantation surgery. *Audiol Neurootol* **21**(4):244–9.
18. Majdani O, Schurzig D, Hussong A, *et al.* (2010) Force measurement of insertion of cochlear implant electrode arrays *in vitro*: Comparison of surgeon to automated insertion tool. *Acta Otolaryngol* **130**(1):31–6.
19. Carlson ML, Driscoll CL, Gifford RH, *et al.* (2011) Implications of minimizing trauma during conventional cochlear implantation. *Otol Neurotol* **32**(6):962–8.
20. Kaufmann CR, Henslee AM, Claussen A, *et al.* (2020) Evaluation of insertion forces and cochlea trauma following robotics-assisted cochlear implant electrode array insertion. *Otol Neurotol* **41**(5):631–8.
21. Zhang, H. (2023). An Intraoperative Force Perception and Signal Decoupling Method on Capsulorhexis Forceps. *arXiv preprint arXiv:2311.07909.*

15 Advocating One's Rights as a Child or Adult With Hearing Loss

Donna L. Sorkin, MA[1]

What Is Self-Advocacy?

Advocacy is an activity undertaken by individuals or groups that aims to influence decisions by government officials or private decision-makers via education, media outreach, and other means. Although there is a perception that someone needs special training or education to advocate, in fact anyone can be an effective advocate. You already have the most important and valuable tool you need: your story or that of your child. No one understands the ins and outs of your needs as a person with hearing loss or a parent or guardian of a child who is deaf and hard of hearing as well as you do.

Self-advocacy is the ability to speak up for yourself. Being an advocate for yourself or your child involves the identification of your needs or your child's needs, your clear delineation of those needs, and your skill in facilitating intervention by others to allow them to understand how they can support you and then follow through with appropriate actions. Self-advocacy is beneficial in all areas of life — from returning a defective purchase to working out solutions with difficult neighbors. The focus of this chapter is on advocacy that may be undertaken by adults for their own needs or by adults on behalf of children who are deaf or hard of hearing and the right to have their communication needs addressed. Such rights are part of our Federal laws that seek to allow people full participation in their life's journey.

Despite what we are entitled to, we may not follow through to pursue solutions that may help us. One of the reasons for not following through relates to perspectives about disability — both our own mindsets about

---

[1] Executive director of the American Cochlear Implant Alliance.

ourselves or our children and societal constructs that drive our thinking about being less than perfect. In the case of hearing loss, we often hear about adults who bluff when they do not hear. Rather than admitting that someone is not following the conversation and asking for a repeat, we may see behaviors that are intended to 'cover' rather than being exposed as not being able to hear. There are also many examples of adults who withdraw from family gatherings and other social events because of their inability to hear and fully participate. This approach to addressing one's hearing issues makes it more difficult to advocate because people have lost confidence in themselves and may not be willing (or able) to step up and ask for the accommodations that they are entitled to.

In a similar (denial) approach, we are sometimes told by parents that their child does so well with their hearing technology that they need no support at school. For such families, the child's excellent progress at learning language becomes a badge of honor and a perspective that their child is now 'normal.' Without noting the psychological and emotional aspects of this kind of thinking and the potential impact on their child, it is important to recognize that the concept of disability and acceptance of the fact that one *has* a disability underlies the framework for our laws that provide access and inclusion in the United States. It is the identification of the disability and the acknowledged limitations that the disability entails that determines eligibility for services and support under our legal system.

Inheriting Hearing Loss

I grew up with hearing loss in my family. Both my father and my paternal grandmother were hard of hearing. Though I never saw her audiogram, I suspect that my grandmother was profoundly deaf. Because hearing technology was considerably less effective during my grandmother's lifetime, combined with the reality that she never learned to lipread well, my grandmother was left out of most conversations. Of course, I loved her but we had little connection. My father's hearing loss was also significant. Although he used hearing aids throughout his adult life, my father's inability to perform essential aspects of his job forced his early retirement at age 52. Remarkably, he never discussed with his children or friends his hearing disability as the health-related reason for leaving a job that he loved . At that time, there was literally no mechanism for providing support in the workplace for someone with hearing loss — even in the Federal government where my father was employed for his entire working life. He struggled on the telephone, in meetings, and at Congressional hearings where one cannot afford to make errors. The stress of not hearing exacerbated other health issues and eventually forced him to retire though he never spoke about the issues that hearing loss caused him at work — even to his own family.

My own situation was very different as I grew up in a timeframe with dramatically improved hearing technology — cochlear implants, digital hearing aids, bone-anchored solutions, and assistive devices for adults and children as well as Federal laws that require public and private institutions to address access and inclusion in the workplace, at school, in public places, and anywhere people wish to go. Through such Federal laws, the United States has dramatically expanded support services for children at school and under early intervention, in public places, and in the telecommunications arena for people of all ages. These changes have made possible a different sort of life for people with hearing loss in a society that now recognizes that equity, inclusion, and accommodation are not only the right thing to do but also the economically smart thing to do. People who work and take care of themselves become contributors rather than individuals who require extensive financial support.[1]

Concept of Disability and Personal Perspectives

In the United States, the concept of full inclusion has evolved from earlier timeframes when we excluded children and adults with disabilities from the mainstream because of a lack of accommodations or sometimes a belief that having a disability made someone less able to participate in employment, school, or cultural activities. In the past, this kind of discrimination sometimes meant that people with disabilities were hidden away in institutional settings. Some families were sometimes embarrassed by having a child who was considered to be 'less whole.' Children with hearing loss were typically educated in special schools and parents who wished to have their children go to mainstream schools often did so with no accommodations and even resistance from the school.

There was (and still is) a perceived stigma associated with hearing loss.[2] Because of that stigma, it was not unusual for people to attempt to hide their hearing loss; this was especially prevalent because the disability is not readily obvious. Even today, many adults and parents of children who are deaf or hard of hearing are hesitant to reveal their hearing loss and because of that, they may decline to utilize technology that could help them. Adults who could benefit from cochlear implants may not opt to pursue one because of the cosmetic aspects of wearing the device. A 2023 survey conducted by American Cochlear Implant Alliance of adults who might benefit from a CI found that 52% of respondents indicated that one of the reasons why they did not go forward was that they were 'concerned about the way the CI looked and its visibility on the head.'[3]

Federal Role in Access for Adults and Children With Disabilities

The environment today is one in which there is an expectation that we will provide accommodations for all who need them. Children and adults with disabilities — including hearing loss — are now living at a time when we accept the fact that society will provide ramps for inclusion whether those ramps are for people with physical constraints, limitations in sight, hearing loss, or any other condition that meets the federal standard of disability.

The Americans with Disabilities Act (ADA) defines an individual with a disability as a person who has a physical or mental impairment that substantially limits one or more major life activities. The four major types of disabilities are categorized as physical, developmental, behavioral or emotional, and sensory. Hearing loss is considered as a sensory disability. The ADA was the first legislation to establish a *comprehensive* prohibition of discrimination on the basis of disability.[4,5]

This is an overview of the concept of self-advocacy and a discussion of Federal laws that may help families — children or adults with hearing loss — to know and be able to access the services and accommodations that they are entitled to under our Federal legal system. Three types of accommodations, important to deaf and hard of hearing people of all ages, are important in our country. These are the services and accommodations provided in laws related to: education, telecommunications, and general access.

Some issues to keep in mind as individuals negotiate the legal support system for children and adults who are deaf and hard of hearing are especially important:

- The passage of laws is only the first step. In general, the laws are in place in the US but ensuring that an adult or child receives those services is another matter entirely.
- Understanding the jargon of the laws is critical to knowing how to negotiate the system. The proverbial alphabet soup of abbreviations and terminology is intimidating — particularly with respect to education laws.
- To be eligible for services, an individual adult or child must acknowledge that they have a hearing loss and need help or need specific services.

Education Laws

There are several Federal laws in the education realm that are relevant. The most frequently cited is the Individuals with Disabilities Education Act, which addresses the educational needs of children. Key elements include:

- *Free and appropriate public education*: School districts are required to provide services and accommodations that meet the specific needs of a child. For a child with a cochlear implant or hearing aid, this might be an frequency modulation (FM) system which filters sound to remove environmental noise and amplify the speaker, captioning or sign interpreters (depending upon the needs of the child), support services such as a teacher of the deaf, note-taking, preferential seating, or acoustical adaptations. Free means families cannot be charged and appropriate means the school must look at the individual child's needs. Services that may be appropriate for a child with a CI might include speech and audiology services or psychological services.
- *Least restrictive environment* (LRE): Federal law supports the concept that children with hearing loss should be educated with children who have typical hearing to the extent possible. LRE can be a source of

controversy when parents and schools disagree on services that should be provided to achieve the LRE. Sometimes the objective is a mainstream placement and sometimes it is something else.

- The process of determining what services are provided occurs via the *Individualized education plan*: It is here that parents need to hone their advocacy skills on behalf of their child(ren). Other professionals on the child's team such as the CI audiologist, speech pathologist, or AVT are often helpful. Parents do not need to go this route alone!

Telecommunication Laws

Before the communication transformation that began in earnest in the mid-1990s with a rollout of digital wireless cell phones with a plethora of features, telecommunications relay services with professional captioners working 24/7 and the development and ongoing expansion of the Internet as society's main communication tool, telecommunications was one of the most limiting aspects of having a hearing loss. These new services made an extraordinary difference in the everyday life of everyone but most especially deaf and hard of hearing people of all ages. The services we take for granted now provide inclusion and equity in a way that my father could never had imagined. Advocates quickly foresaw the potential and moved to include consideration of access of users of hearing aids and cochlear implants in the design of technology and the provision of services. Perhaps the most important law in this category was Section 255 of the Telecommunications Act of 1996, which required that *telecommunications products and services be accessible to, and usable by, people with disabilities, if readily achievable.*[6] The legislation was remarkable in that it brought attention, for the first time, to the diverse communication needs of the population. This requirement that closed captioning of all television programming was a watershed for people with a range of needs. As time went on, captioning became commonplace everywhere and is now used by people with, and without, hearing loss.

General Access

The ADA, passed in 1990, was intended to protect people with disabilities from discrimination in all aspects of their lives. When my father retired from his job in 1971 because he could not perform essential aspects of his employment, there were no accommodations for his hearing loss. Indeed, he had no idea what might help him. Twenty years later, when I testified in front of Congress on issues related to hearing aid provision, I used an assistive listening device that allowed me to hear and understand the questions posed to me by Senators in the noisy, reverberant hearing room. My mother, who never demonstrated any interest in my work, asked if she could attend. Later, while talking about the Congressional hearing, I asked her why she had requested to come and she shared 'I wanted to see you do what your father could not.'

> *The ADA raised the bar for what was expected to be provided to people with disabilities in four key areas of everyday life: employment; state- and local government-provided programs including recreation and social services; public accommodations covering anywhere people go including restaurants, doctors' offices, hotels, stores, theatres, and private schools; and telecommunications relay services.*

Owning One's Hearing Loss

Proactively tackling one's hearing loss or supporting a child along their journey begins with pursuing hearing technology or other therapies that are appropriate. Some may choose to utilize a visual communication mode such as ASL or Cued Speech. Self-advocacy also means that we recognize that hearing loss often changes over time, just as one's life circumstances change over time. Recognizing that there is a continuum of hearing care solutions and staying abreast of information that can help someone pursue the right solution along that continuum at the right time is critical to the partnership between patients and hearing care providers.

This chapter provides encouragement for adults with hearing loss and parents of children who are deaf or hard of hearing to practice self-advocacy to benefit from the wide-ranging laws that exist today and provide opportunities that can help children and adults to take advantage of all that life has to offer. These are basic rights in America that are provided for in national legislation. Learn what is available and develop the skills to negotiate the system. There is so much more opportunity today for people who are deaf and hard of hearing, given the vastly improved hearing technology and the laws that provide the accommodations and services that adults and children need to fully participate.

References

1. Cheng AK, Rubin HR, Powe NR, *et al.* (2000) Cost utility of the cochlear implant in children. *JAMA* **284**(7):850–6.
2. David D, Werner P. (2022) Stigma regarding hearing loss and hearing aids: A scoping review. *Stigma Health* **1**(2):59–71.
3. Sorkin DL. (2023) Adult Perceptions of Hearing Status and Options. AudiologyOnline.
4. Americans with Disabilities Act of 1990, 42 U.S.C. § 12101 et seq. (1990).
5. Livability Magazine. (2015 August 14) A Brief History of Disability Rights & The Americans with Disabilities Act. https://ability360.org/livability/advocacy-livability/history-disability-rights-ada/ (accessed on 2023 August 23).
6. Federal Communications Commission. (1996) The Telecommunications Act of 1996 and People with Disabilities. https://www.fcc.gov/general/telecommunications-act-1996-and-people-disabilities (accessed on 2023 September 9).

Helpful Resources

ADA.gov, US Department of Justice. (2020) *Guide to Disability Rights Laws.* https://www.ada.gov/resources/disability-rights-guide (accessed on 2023 August 23).

American Cochlear Implant Alliance. (2021) Advocating for Cochlear Implant Access: ACI Alliance Toolkit for Action. https://www.acialliance.org/page/AdvocacyToolkit

Siegel Attorney LM. (2023) *Complete IEP Guide: How to Advocate for Your Special Ed Child.* NOLO.

Sorkin DL. (2019) Education and access laws for children with hearing loss. In: Madell JR, Flexer C, Wolfe J, Schafer EC (eds.), *Pediatric Audiology: Diagnosis, Technology, and Management* (3rd ed.). Thieme. https://www.acialliance.org/page/lawschildrenhearingloss

Glossary

Acute otitis media: Recent onset of infection of the middle ear space, most common in children, but can also occur in adults.

Adenoids: Lymphoid tissues located at the back of the nasal passage.

Air-conduction hearing threshold: Measurement of hearing threshold of stimuli presented through the air, using audiometric equipment.

Alport syndrome: Rare genetic disorder involving type IV collagen which presents with deafness, visual abnormalities, and kidney disease.

Anamnesis: A patient's account of medical history.

Atelectatic otitis: Retraction of the ear drum secondary to chronic infection, inflammation, or eustachian tube dysfunction.

Atherosclerosis: Deposition of plaques in the inner walls of arteries which can obstruct blood flow.

Auditory evoked brainstem responses (ABRs): Objective measurement of auditory pathway function from the inner ear to the brain. Used in patients who are unable to undergo traditional audiometry or who are suspected to have auditory nerve pathology.

Autoimmune inner ear disease (AIED): Bilateral (sometimes unilateral) sensorineural hearing loss secondary to an inappropriate immune response that targets the patient's own hearing structures.

Barotrauma: Injury secondary to changes in air pressure. It can occur during diving, flying, and hyperbaric therapy.

The Glossary is the work of Jaimee Cooper, BS and Adrien A. Eshraghi MD, MSc, FACS.

Bone-conduction hearing thresholds: A hearing test in which the ability to hear sound transmitted via bone to the cochlea is determined. For example, bone conduction thresholds are decreased when there is damage to ossicles or a perforation of the ear drum.

Bony labyrinth: Rigid, bony structure that covers the inner ear structures, including semicircular canals, cochlea, and vestibule.

Branchio-oto-renal syndrome: A genetic condition characterized by branchial fistulae, ear malformations causing hearing loss, and renal malformations.

Central auditory processing disorder (CAPD): A spectrum of diseases (also known as auditory processing disorders) which impact the processing of auditory information between the auditory nerve to the brain, but the inner, middle, and outer ear are functioning appropriately.

Cerumen: Ear wax.

CHARGE syndrome: A disorder which is characterized by coloboma, heart defects, atresia choanae, renal abnormalities, genital abnormalities, growth retardation, and ear abnormalities that causes hearing loss.

Cholesteatoma: A benign tumor of the ear that is formed by a collection of skin debris that grows and can destroy surrounding structures. It can cause hearing loss and eardrum perforation. If untreated and very advanced, dizziness, facial paralysis, and even brain and neck abscess may occur.

Chronic otitis media: Longstanding or recurrent middle ear infection or inflammation with or without the presence of a TM perforation which may lead to hearing loss.

Chronic suppurative otitis media: Persistent ear infection/inflammation typically with an ear drum perforation which leads to chronic draining of the ear and hearing loss.

Clinical trial: Studies in humans which seek to test the safety and efficacy of new treatments. After animal testing is complete, they begin with testing the treatment safety and appropriate dosage on a small group of healthy individuals (Phase 1). Then efficacy and side effects are determined with a small group of individuals with the disease (Phase 2), followed by a larger group of individuals with the disease to determine efficacy compared to existing treatment (Phase 3). After Phase 3, the treatment must go through FDA approval, once approved it enters post market surveillance which looks for long term side effects (Phase 4).

Cochlea: A fluid filled spiral shaped structure located within the temporal bone that constitutes the inner ear. It contains the sensory cells to allow for hearing.

Cochlear implant: A prostatic hearing device for individuals with SNHL which is surgically placed with its electrode in the cochlea that allows for electrical stimulation of the auditory nerve thus restoring some hearing function.

Conductive hearing loss (CHL): Hearing loss that is due to ineffective or absent transduction of sound from the external environment to the cochlea, through the external and middle ear.

Cribriform plate: A thin bone which separates the cranial fossa and the nasal cavity.

Decibel (dB): A unit of measurement for sound intensity, it is a logarithmic scale.

Dura: The outer most soft tissue covering of the brain just below the skull.

Electroacoustic devices: Hearing devices which combine the use of electrical stimulation (cochlear implant) and acoustic devices (hearing aid) to restore hearing.

Endocochlear potential: It is related to the differing electrolyte composition of the endolymph and perilymph in the inner ear, cochlea. It is around +80mV. It is involved in the pathomechanism of hearing in which the electrical gradient, and movement of electrolytes, allows for the creation of neural impulses.

Endogenous: Originating from within an organism.

Endolymph: A physiologic fluid, comprised of potassium, as the major cation, and sodium. It is found in the Scala media where the sensory cells of hearing and organ of Corti are located in the cochlea.

Endolymphatic Duct: A small anatomical duct that regulates endolymph flow between the vestibular, auditory compartment, and the dura in the intercranial space.

Eustachian tube (ET): A duct that connects the middle ear to the back of the nasal passage, nasopharynx. It helps to maintain the pressure in the middle ear and help to avoid barotrauma.

Exogenous: Originating from outside an organism.

Exostoses: Small benign, bony outgrowths of the ear canal.

External auditory canal: The passageway which sound travels through that connects the external environment to the tympanic membrane.

Frequency: The number of times a sound pressure wave repeats its self per second.

Hearing aid: An external device worn on the outer ear or within the ear canal which consists of a microphone, amplifier, and a speaker.

Helicotrema: The most apical portion of the cochlea where the Scala tympani and Scala vestibuli meet.

Hyperbaric oxygenation: The use of a chamber to increase the ambient oxygen pressure for treatment. Can be used to aid wound healing as it increases the oxygen content of the environment. It can also increase the vascularization of the inner ear and has been proposed as a treatment modality for sudden hearing loss.

Hypoxia: A state of decreased oxygenation of tissues.

Immune-mediated inner ear disease (IMED): Sensorineural hearing loss secondary to immune causes, may include hearing loss and/or vestibular symptoms.

Inner Ear: The innermost portion of the hearing system consisting of the cochlea and vestibular structures.

Inner hair cells (IHC): Sensory cells within the organ of Corti which act at the sensory receptors for auditory information and transmit information to the brain via the auditory nerve.

Lymphocytes: An immune cell that is found in the blood and created in the bone marrow. It comprises 20–45% of the white blood cells in the body. It is increased in times of infection and functions to create antibodies, kill virus infected cells and tumor cells, and regulates immune response. This class of cell includes T cells, B cells, and NK cells.

Macrophages: An immune cell that is responsible for removing pathogens, cellular debris, cancer cells, dead tissues, and any other foreign particles.

Membranous labyrinth: The system of ducts and chambers that reside inside of the bony labyrinth, and contains the endolymph and perilymph of the auditory and vestibular systems.

Meniere's disease: A chronic disorder involving hearing and vestibular symptoms (hearing loss, tinnitus, and vertigo) which is hypothesized to be related to a high pressure of endolymph. The precise etiology is largely unknown but has been proposed to be due to immune, viral, allergic, or inflammatory causes.

Meningitis: Inflammation of the covering membranes of the brain, which is most commonly due to viral or bacterial causes. It can result in hearing loss, by spread of the infection to the inner ear.

Middle Ear: The portion of the auditory system spanning from the ear drum to the round window of the cochlea and includes the ossicles.

Mixed hearing loss (MHL): Hearing loss involving both conductive and sensorineural components.

Modiolus: The bony center of the cochlea which contains the auditory spiral ganglia.

Mondini syndrome: A congenital form of hearing loss where the cochlea has 1.5 turns instead of the normal 2 turns.

Myringoplasty: A procedure whereby a ear drum perforation is closed with a graft from another part of the body (usually temporalis fascia or ear cartilage) or synthetic material.

Nasopharyngeal: Relating to the most superior area of the pharynx (throat) located posterior to the nose.

Neoplasm: An abnormal growth of tissue (tumor) that can be benign or malignant.

Noise-induced hearing loss (NIHL): Hearing loss secondary to prolonged exposure to loud sound or sudden exposure to very loud sound which damages the sensitive neural structures in the cochlea.

Organ of Corti: A structure in the cochlea which converts mechanical sound waves into neural impulses. It contains the OHCs, IHCs, supporting cells, tectorial membrane, space of nuel, tunnel of Corti, and the basilar membrane.

Ossicles (ossicular chain): The three bones of the middle ear, the malleus, incus, and stapes which conduct sound from the ear drum to the cochlea. They are the smallest bones in the human body.

Osteomas: Growths of bone, which typically grow off of another bone it can be seen in the ear canal, causing obstruction of the canal.

Otalgia: Ear pain.

Otitis media: Inflammation of the middle ear, usually due to infection.

Otolith: Small crystals comprised of calcium carbonate located in the vestibular system of the inner ear, which allow humans to detect acceleration, linear, and rotational movement in space.

Otorrhagia: Bleeding from the ear.

Otorrhea: Drainage from the ear.

Otosclerosis: A condition involving commonly ossification of the ossicular chain resulting in conductive hearing loss. It is most common in females and may worsen with pregnancy. It can also effect the inner ear (cochlea), causing a mixed or sensorineural hearing loss.

Otoscopy: A clinical procedure which looks into the external ear canal to appreciate the ear drum, external ear canal. The clinician can appreciate some abnormalities of the middle ear space (fluid, cholesteatoma).

Ototoxicity: Inner ear damage secondary to local or systemic medications.

Outer Ear: Consists of the pinna and the opening to the external ear canal. The pinna includes the helix, antihelix, and tragus.

Outer hair cells (OHC): Cells within the organ of Corti which act to fine tune the frequency and sensitivity of the vibrations within the cochlea. They connect to efferent nerves which originate in the brain. There are three rows of outer hair cells.

Pendred syndrome: A genetic disease which presents as bilateral hearing loss and goiter, which is enlargement of the thyroid gland.

Perilymph: Physiologic fluid within the Scala tympany and Scala vestibuli. The electrochemical gradient between endolymph and perilymph allows for the organ of Corti to function as the hearing organ.

Perimodiolar: A specific variety of cochlear implant electrode arrays; these are designed to sit against the modiolus placing it in closer contact with the nerve fibers in the cochlea.

Permanent threshold shift (PTS): Changes in hearing thresholds after noise trauma which do not return to normal with time, as opposed to temporary threshold shifts which return to normal over time.

Phenotype: The observable characteristics of an organism, results from a combination of their genotype and environmental interactions.

Plasma cells: An immune cell derived from B lymphocytes which produce antibodies, they are essential for humoral immunity.

Presbycusis: Age-related hearing loss.

Pure-tone audiometry: The gold standard test for assessing hearing. It is a subjective, behavioral test which involves a patient responding (usually with a button press) to stimuli at different frequencies (pitches).

Reissner's membrane: The dividing membrane between the Scala vestibuli and the Scala media. It allows for nutrients to pass between the endolymph and perilymph, and may be involved in the pathogenesis of Meniere's disease.

Retroauricular: Pertaining to the area behind the ear.

Round window: A membrane covered orifice on the cochlea which acts to decompress the pressure from fluid waves created by the stapes vibrating on the oval window after they have traveled through the cochlea. It can be utilized to deliver drugs to the inner ear (cochlea) for therapeutic benefit.

Saccule: A component on the vestibular system which detects linear motion in the vertical plane. It contains vestibular hair cells and otoliths.

Scala media: It is in the cochlea contains endolymph and the organ of Corti.

Scala tympani: A perilymph filled duct within the cochlea. This is the space that cochlear implant electrodes are inserted and is commonly accessed via the round window. It is separated from the Scala media by the basilar membrane. At the helicotrema it becomes the scala vestibuli (also known as the vestibular duct).

Scala vestibuli: A perilymph filled duct which communicates with the Scala tympani an the helicotrema. It is separated from the Scala media by Reissner's membrane.

Schwannomas: Tumors derived from the supporting cells of the peripheral nervous system known as Schwann cells. Common schwannomas are found on the eighth cranial nerve known as vestibular schwannomas (acoustic neuromas). They can cause hearing loss or dizziness.

Semicircular canal dehiscence: Thinning of the bony capsule of the semicircular canals.

Semicircular canals: The portion of the vestibular system which detects rotational/angular motion and acceleration. It is comprised of three canals, lateral, anterior, and posterior, each responsible for movement around the vertical, lateral, and anterio-posterior axes, respectively.

Sensorineural hearing loss (SNHL): Hearing loss that is due to damage of the neural structures in the cochlea or auditory nerve. Can be due to genetic, traumatic noise, or age-related causes.

Stereocilia: Thin hair like protrusion found within sensory organs (i.e. cochlea, vestibular system). They are the mechanosensors which respond to the motion of the perilymph in the cochlea and vestibular apparatus.

Stria vascularis: The small capillaries which help to perfuse and transmit nutrients and oxygen to the structures in the organ of Corti, it is found on the lateral wall of the cochlea.

Sudden sensorineural hearing loss (SSNHL): Sensorineural hearing loss of 30dB or greater over a maximum of 72 hours. This form of hearing loss may be initially and aggressively treated with systemic or intra-tympanic local steroids which can help reverse the hearing loss in many cases.

Synaptopathies: Disorders which arise from defects in synaptic communication between hair cells its accompanying nerve that takes information to the brain.

Tectorial membrane: Also known as Reissner's membrane. It is an acellular membrane that spans the length of the organ of Corti and moves in response to vibrations of the perilymph. This movement allows for transmission of electrical signals by the inner hair cells which is received by the brain as auditory information.

Temporary threshold shifts (TTS): Changes in hearing thresholds after noise trauma which return to normal within a few days.

Tinnitus: Perception of sound in the absence of an external source. Tinnitus can be peripheral (within the cochlea) or central (within the brain). Tinnitus that begins peripherally, can 'centralize' over the course of 1–2 years if not resolved.

Tonotopic: Organization whereby specific sound frequencies are received by specific receptors. The cochlea has a tonotopic organization, the most basal portion detects high frequency stimuli and the apical portion detects low frequency stimuli.

Tympanic atelectasis: Retraction and/or atrophy of the tympanic membrane, usually secondary to infection or inflammation.

Tympanic membrane: The separation of the external and middle ears. It converts and amplifies air vibrations form the environment into mechanical vibrations of the ossicular chain.

Tympanometry: A diagnostic test which uses air pressure to determine the functioning of the tympanic membrane and the state of the middle ear.

Usher syndrome: An inherited genetic condition which involves both hearing loss and visual defects.

Utricle: A component on the vestibular system which detects linear motion in the horizontal plane. It contains vestibular hair cells and otoliths.

Vertigo: A sensation of motion or spinning of vestibular origin.

Vestibular rehabilitation therapy (VRT): Specialized therapy used in patients with vestibular symptoms (dizziness or imbalance) to retrain the brain and help reestablish vestibular function. It helps to improve eye, ear, and cerebellar coordination.

Vestibular system: The portions of the inner ear which provides a sense of balance and inform the brain on body position, in conjunction with the eyes, cerebellum, and brain. It is comprised of the semicircular canals, utricle, and saccule and works closely with the cochlea.

Vestibule: The central portion of the bony labyrinth that contains the utricle and saccule.

Waardenburg syndrome: A genetic condition which presents with hearing loss and light skin, hair, and eyes. Additionally, patients may have a widened nasal bridge.

Index

www.ingramcontent.com/pod-product-compliance
Lightning Source LLC
LaVergne TN
LVHW010033160826
845671LV00004B/187
* 9 7 8 9 8 1 1 2 8 7 9 6 1 *